Acknowledgements

Assessment Task Force

Marybell Avery

Ben Dyson

Jennifer L. Fisette

Connie Fox

Marian Franck

Kim C. Graber

Judith H. Placek, chair

Judith Rink

Weimo Zhu

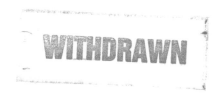

Technical Assistance

Connie Fox

Pamela MacFarlane

Youngsik Park

De Raynes, Senior Manager for Physical Education

Charlene Burgeson, Executive Director

NASPE would like to extend its appreciation to the many professionals who served as Project Administrators and coders in the gathering of thousands of pieces of individual student data for the Elementary Standard 1 assessments. This list includes:

Ginger Aaron, Beverly Allen, Marybell Avery, Sherry Baggett-McMinn, Dominique Banville, Martie Bell, Debra Berkey, Carol Blair, Heidi Bohler, Mary Buddemeier, Eric Carpenter, Nancy Christensen, Catherine Conte, Mary Cramer, Judy Cunningham, Char Darst, Ben Dyson, Ellen Eisman, Joyce Ellis, Robert Emery, Heather Erwin, Matt Evans, John Ferguson, Hugh Ferry, Jennifer Fisette, Connie Fox, Marian Franck, Rodney Fry, Ovande Furtado, Ritchie Gabbei, Jere Gallagher, Caecilia Gropp, Mary Ann Guinn, Cindy Haigh, Tarin Hampton, Vanessa Hardbarger, Brent Heidron, Cindy Heos, Pat Hewitt, Lisa Hicks, Kathy Hixon, Kath Howarth, Becky Hull, Susan Jackson, Arcelia Jeffreys, Berniece Jones, Sherman Jones, Stephanie Jones, Pat Jordan, Susan Jordan, Michael Judd, Pam Keese, Barbi Kelley, Ulrike Kerstges, Kym Kirby, Tony Kirk, Gray Komich, Brenda Knitter, Toni Leo, Brenda Lichtman, Cindy Lins, Sue Long, Bob Martin, Carol Martini, Koji Matsushima, Marguerite McDonald, Shaunna McGhie, Chad McLarty, Beverly Nichols, Amber Phillips, Molly Pickering, Virginia Politano, Linda Poor, Penny Portman, Lisa Pryor, De Raynes, Suzanne Reed, Karen Roof, Patrice Scharin, Charlie Schmidt, Jan Scott, Eugenia Scott, Deborah Sheehey, Sally Smallwood, Kate Splendore, Susan Stewart, Marilyn Sting, Pat Stueck, Ann-Catherine Sullivan, Charmain Sutherland, Cetan Tameris, Sue Tarr, Jackie Thompson, Jen Thompson, Steve Underwood, Emily Vall, Mindy Welch, Sharon Welch, Carol Winckler, Nanette Wolford, Cheryl Wyatt

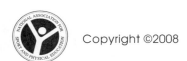 Copyright ©2008

National Association for Sport and Physical Education

an association of the American Alliance for Health, Physical Education,
Recreation and Dance.

Address orders to AAHPERD Publications, P.O. Box 385, Oxon Hill, MD 20750-0385, call 1.800.321.0789 or order online
at www.naspeinfo.org. Order item 304-10458.

ISBN: 978-0-88314-930-0

Printed in the United States of America.

T able of Contents

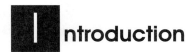

Introduction

Standards-Based Education

Since the late 1980s education reform in the United States has been largely driven by setting academic standards that describe what students should know and are able to do, and the development of accountability systems for measuring student achievement of the standards. Terms such as "standards-based education", "standards-based educational reform" and "standards movement" are common in today's education vernacular.

Standards and assessment have been pivotal themes in recent reform efforts, cutting across much of the federal legislation passed by Congress to improve the education of all students. Standards-based education began in 1994 when Congress passed *Goals 2000: Educate America Act*. This established a framework which identified world-class academic standards, measured student progress and provided the support for any student needing help in meeting the standards. The Act codified into law eight national education goals: school readiness, school completion, student achievement and citizenship, teacher education and professional development, mathematics and science, adult literacy and lifelong learning, alcohol- and drug-free schools and parental participation.

Since the implementation of Goals 2000, the *Elementary and Secondary School Education Act of 1965* (ESEA) has been amended or reauthorized twice. In 1994, the *Improving America's Schools Act* focused on changing the way education is delivered, encouraging comprehensive school reform, upgrading instructional and professional development to align with high standards, strengthening accountability and promoting the coordination of resources to improve education for all children.

The most recent reauthorization of ESEA, the *No Child Left Behind Act of 2001* (NCLB) addresses increased accountability for states, school districts and schools, greater choice for parents and students (particularly those attending low-performing schools), more flexibility for state and local education agencies in the use of federal education dollars and a stronger emphasis on reading, (especially for our youngest children). Together these federal laws have established many of the principles of standards-based reform, including the expectation that *all* students will attain high standards of academic excellence.

Standards-based education requires clear, measurable standards for all students. Standards and benchmarks identify what students should know and be able to do as they progress through school and should be written so they are developmentally appropriate and relevant to future education and employment needs. They also should be written so that all students are capable of achieving them and talented students will exceed them.

Standards are meant to be anchors, aligning curriculum, instruction and assessment. This explains the emergence of the terms "standards-based curriculum", "standards-based instruction", and "standards-based assessment" as well as the holistic term, "standards-based education". By design, standards-based education lends itself to accountability.

Standards-Based Accountability

In years past, education accountability was conducted by measuring school inputs and processes such as funding levels, curriculum offering and resources and regulation compliance. After the development of national and state standards, policymakers began to shift the focus of accountability to student outcomes. Now policymakers are emphasizing student learning and achievement outcomes to gauge the success of the education system. This trend in education reform is known as standards-based accountability. Systems have been and continue to be put into place to hold states, districts, schools and teachers accountable for the performance of their students.

Standards-based accountability systems use criterion-referenced performance standards rather than norm-referenced rankings. A standards-based system measures each student against the concrete standard, instead of measuring how well a student performs when compared to others.

Once standards are established, the next step in building a standards-based accountability system is the alignment of curriculum to the standards. The specific knowledge or skills which students must acquire to meet the standards must be defined and criterion-referenced assessments must be established to determine the extent to which students meet the standards. The alignment of instruction and formative assessment of the standards must follow.

Standards-Based Education and Accountability for Physical Education

The National Association for Sport and Physical Education (NASPE) has established itself as a leader in standards-based education. In 1995, NASPE published *Moving into the Future: National Standards for Physical Education* followed by a second edition in 2004.

The National Standards for Physical Education state that "physical activity is critical to the development and maintenance of good health. The goal of physical education is to develop physically educated individuals who have the knowledge, skills and confidence to enjoy a lifetime of healthful physical activity" (NASPE, 2004). A physically educated person is defined by these six standards.

1. Demonstrates competency in motor skills and movement patterns needed to perform a variety of physical activities.
2. Demonstrates understanding of movement concepts, principles, strategies and tactics as they apply to the learning and performance of physical activities.
3. Participates regularly in physical activity.
4. Achieves and maintains a health-enhancing level of physical fitness.
5. Exhibits responsible personal and social behavior that respects self and others in physical activity settings.
6. Values physical activity for health, enjoyment, challenge, self-expression, and/or social interaction.

The national standards are presented in grade-level ranges representing grades K-2, 3-5, 6-8 and 9-12 so that ranges are consistent with developmental patterns of children and youth, reflect organizational patterns in public school settings and align with other content areas. Each grade-level range contains two sections: student expectations and sample performance outcomes. The student expectations reflect what students should know and are able to do at the end of each grade-level range (e.g., K-2). The sample performance outcomes are examples of student behavior at each grade-level range that demonstrate progress toward achieving the standards. Until now, the missing element of standards-based physical education has been the absence of nationally tested assessments and rubrics to measure student achievement of the national standards and benchmarks.

With the publication of *PE Metrics: Assessing the National Standards* (NASPE, 2008), the gap has been closed. *PE Metrics* provides valid and reliable standards-based assessments and rubrics ("NASPE assessments") to measure student achievement of the national standards by high school graduation and appropriate progress at three other grade-level ranges. The assessments give evidence of learning through student work/performance while the rubrics describe the quality of the work/performance. Teachers and schools have the ability to report student progress on each standard using a rubric that describes various levels of knowledge and skills. The advantage to this approach is that it provides students, teachers and parents with highly specific information.

It is critical to align curriculum instruction and assessments with one another and with state and national standards. To provide students with a truly standards-based physical education, teachers must be certain the material on which students are being assessed aligns with what is being taught in class. Assessment as part of the instructional process is much more than evaluation and accountability. Teachers should use a variety of techniques including the NASPE assessments as part of regular classroom instruction. Assessment integrated with instruction (e.g. pre-assessment and formative assessment) is imperative for maximizing student learning and success. It is equally important to use pre-assessment and formative assessment to communicate to students important skills and knowledge and to properly prepare students for summative assessment. For accountability purposes, it isn't necessary to assess all students on every task; a random sample of student performance can be used to guide curriculum development or to report on programmatic success to administration or district leaders.

National Association for Sport and Physical Education, an association of the American Alliance for Health, Physical Education, Recreation and Dance

3

4

National Association for Sport and Physical Education, an association of the American Alliance for Health, Physical Education, Recreation and Dance

Overview of the NASPE Assessment Project

The National Association for Sport and Physical Education (NASPE) is committed to the tenets of quality physical education, which include the opportunity for all children to learn through supportive policies and environment (e.g., certified teachers, adequate facilities and equipment), national standards, quality curriculum, appropriate instructional practices and student and program assessment. NASPE continues to develop tools to help schools, districts and states implement assessments measuring student achievement of state and national physical education standards. As the only national association for physical education, NASPE feels a strong obligation to develop valid and reliable assessments that can be used by teachers throughout the nation.

In March 1999, NASPE assembled a "think tank" of university and public school professionals to consider how to best advance K-12 physical education. The group was charged with recommending a plan of action to confront the barriers to high quality physical education. The development of performance indicators and practical assessments to evaluate student achievement of the national standards for physical education was the priority recommendation.

In January 2000, NASPE identified experts in physical education to lead what became known as the Assessment Task Force, made up of curriculum and instruction researchers, measurement and evaluation experts, teacher educators, K-12 physical education teachers, administrators and students. It was charged with developing performance indicators corresponding to the national standards at each grade-level range (K-2, 3-5, 6-8, and 9-12) and assessments for each indicator. The performance indicators were not meant to be a comprehensive set of all possible skills and knowledge students should master in a specific grade-level range, but rather samples of performance that could be expected within the grade-level range.

Performance Indicator and Assessment Development

Just as it was not feasible to identify all possible performance indicators, it became clear to the task force that it would not be feasible to write all possible assessments for each indicator. The NASPE examples illustrate good assessment that also serve to guide teachers, districts and states in developing additional assessments.

Ultimately, the task force identified a broad range of performance indicators and wrote a variety of assessments to measure student skills and knowledge. The draft performance indicators and assessments were first introduced to approximately 220 professionals attending a session at the 2001 American Alliance for Health, Physical Education, Recreation and Dance (AAHPERD) National Convention. NASPE continues to update the indicators and assessments project and solicit member feedback during each year's AAHPERD National Convention as well as other relevant conferences.

Institutional Review Board Approval

In preparation for data collection, NASPE obtained Institutional Review Board (IRB) approval for the use of human subjects in a research study from the University of Illinois at Urbana-Champaign (UIUC) and Northern Illinois University (NIU). IRB approval was obtained in 2003 and has been renewed each year, as required by federal law. Although the IRB was written to enable project administrators from different universities to use the same consent documents, the project administrators were advised to make sure UIUC IRB approval would satisfy the IRB requirements at their home institution. In the end, all project administrators submitted joint agreements with UIUC or were covered under the NIU IRB.

Data Collectors

NASPE trained teacher educators to supervise administration of the pilot and oversee the national data collection. These project administrators were chosen based on four criteria: (1) they had established contacts with teachers and administrators in the public schools through their placements of pre-service students for field experience, (2) they had experience with video taping student performances, (3) they had knowledge of the appropriate execution of motor skills, and (4) their research background meant they understood the importance of strict adherence to testing protocols, such as obtaining school district permission and parent/student consent for testing, as well as following the exact assessment description and instructions, including equipment, site preparation, safety and video-taping. Project administrators were recruited through personal contacts made by NASPE staff and task force members and received six hours of training which included a history and overview of the project, roles and responsibilities (including gaining entry, informed consent, videotaping and coding), protocols for videotaping and conducting the assessments, typical videotaping problems and coding video records guidelines. Training took place at the AAHPERD National Convention (2004, 2005, 2006, 2007) and regional and district conferences (2004, 2007).

Process for Testing and Data Collection

Each assessment was subjected to the following sequence of testing: pre-pilot data collection, pilot data collection and national data collection.

Pre-pilot Data Collection

All assessments were pre-piloted by at least one elementary teacher and 20 students. Teachers completed a form requesting feedback of assessment instructions for teachers and students, camera placement and difficulty of assessment task. The assessments were revised based on this feedback along with feedback from a 2003 AAHPERD National Convention session. During the same period as the pre-pilot, the national standards for physical education were reduced from seven to six; therefore, both the performance indicators and assessments had to be modified to meet the new standards and grade-level ranges. Accordingly, some additional pre-pilot feedback was collected.

Pilot Data Collection

Assessments were then tested on a larger scale to further ensure their appropriateness and to collect preliminary data on discrimination validity and reliability. Data was collected from various parts of the country through an extensive network of project administrators.

Each pilot assessment was completed by at least forty students. Project administrators collected parent/student/teacher consent forms, worked with an elementary physical education teacher to administer the assessments and video-recorded, coded, and provided feedback on the assessments. The data were analyzed to make sure the assessments were appropriately difficult and revealed meaningful differences among students. The task force revised the assessments as needed based on data analysis and the feedback from teachers and project administrators.

National Data Collection

Data collection began in February 2005 and continued through winter 2007-2008. The IRB approval from UIUC continued to cover national data collection. An additional IRB was requested and approved from

Northern Illinois University during 2007 and 2008 to cover a subset of data collectors not originally named in the UIUC IRB. See Table 1 for the list of assessments for which national data was collected.

Project administrators collected data from a minimum of 200 students for every assessment task. Two common tasks of medium difficulty were identified at each grade-level range and all students at each grade-level range completed at least one of the two common tasks. The common tasks for Standard 1 elementary assessments were: hopping and dribble with hand (Kindergarten); dribble & jog and jump forward (2nd grade); soccer dribble, pass, and receive, and strike with a paddle (5th grade). The data from the common tasks were used in the research processes to allow scores to be placed on a common scale. This was important in order to be able to equate assessments across and within grade-level ranges and to create an assessment bank.

National Association for Sport and Physical Education, an association of the American Alliance for Health, Physical Education, Recreation and Dance

7

U se of the NASPE Assessments

In today's educational climate there is no place in the school curriculum for a program area that can neither define the outcomes students should achieve nor measure the extent to which students have achieved those outcomes. Too many physical education programs have largely avoided doing both. The instructional process is said to be one of planning or defining outcomes, teaching to achieve those outcomes, and assessing the extent to which students have mastered those outcomes. Physical educators have too often felt that assessment "takes time away from instruction" and failed to recognize that assessment is a very critical part of instruction.

The national standards have provided programs with a guide to determine the critical outcomes of physical education. The NASPE assessment materials provide grade-level range performance indicators and related assessments. Good physical education programs must measure student performance related to meeting the indicators and achieving the standards.

The NASPE assessment materials are intended to be used at different levels for a variety of purposes. Teachers, schools, school district administrators, local, state and national policy makers, and researchers will find them useful in different ways.

Teachers

Teachers use both formative and summative assessment as part of the instructional process. The NASPE assessment materials facilitate both types of assessment. While formative assessment is conducted during the learning process, summative assessment is usually conducted after instruction and is used to determine the results of the instructional process. For example, a formative assessment might be conducted during the middle of a basketball unit to determine if students are learning to dribble correctly. Summative assessment would be conducted at the end of the unit and might assess whether students can dribble and successfully pass the ball without traveling.

Formative assessment. Formative assessment is used to determine skill level prior to and early in the instruction phase. It is not uncommon for teachers to make inaccurate assumptions about the abilities of students in their planning. Using assessment to determine student abilities prior to planning can make instruction far more appropriate. Assessing students prior to planning a unit allows a teacher to compare the results of assessment conducted prior to the unit with that conducted at the end of a unit (summative assessment). This is often referred to as pre- and post-assessment and facilitates a teacher's ability to determine how much students have learned as a result of instruction.

A critical role of formative assessment is its use as a learning experience. Assessment tools can be used to motivate students, set personal goals, analyze performance and clarify expectations for learning. Assessments can also be used to help students and teachers "track" performance over time.

Summative assessment. Valid and reliable assessment tools are critical to summative assessment. Teachers should use valid and reliable assessments in order to determine the effectiveness of instruction and student grades. Reports sent to parents and policy makers on student achievement should be based on objective data. The NASPE assessments are ideally suited for these purposes as they are targeted to the outcomes of instruction appropriate for different grade-level ranges.

District Administrators

The NASPE assessment materials have many potential uses at the school district level. A district can more effectively help students meet physical education standards by graduation if assessment data is used to track the progress of students as they move through the K-12 program. For example, elementary, middle and high school programs can become better aligned with one another and districts can standardize expectations for students across grades and schools. Used this way, assessment can be utilized to improve curriculum planning.

Many physical education programs have functioned without accountability for student learning because there has been no systematic way to measure teacher effectiveness and little effort to measure student performance. Accountability does not limit good programs and teachers; rather, it enhances them. With accountability systems in place, students are provided with feedback on their level of performance and learning and parents are provided with information about their child's progress. Assessment data allows schools and districts to track student achievement, evaluate curricular needs and promote program improvement. Through assessment and accountability physical education takes its place as a critical part of the overall school program. However, a lack of accountability can protect poor programs and ineffective teachers. Districts will find valid and reliable assessments essential for conducting quality physical education programs that produce graduates who value physical activity and have the knowledge and skills to continue to be active adults.

Local, State and National Policy Makers

Consciously or unconsciously, physical educators often overstate what their programs do for children. The field of physical education has claimed much but provided little evidence that it can deliver these promises to their students. Policy makers at all levels want to know if the resources they put into a program have any impact on students. Physical education programs in some areas of the country have recently been "cut" to provide more time for other academic subjects. Without good assessment data, it is difficult to advocate that physical education programs can have an impact on both the traditional goals of our programs and current national health problems.

With the NASPE assessment materials, policy makers will have tools to determine the impact of physical education programs, assess student knowledge and skills in terms of program goals, track student progress over time, compare the quality of programs across districts and states, and provide a way to hold teachers, schools, districts and states responsible for assessing outcomes and meeting program goals.

Researchers

Research on curriculum and instruction in physical education has been hampered by a lack of valid and reliable tools to assess student outcomes. A considerable amount of the research conducted on teaching, teachers, and curriculum in physical education has been related to the processes of teaching without attending to the products of those processes. It is critical the physical education profession is able to identify how to provide students with the skills, knowledge and dispositions they need to lead a physically active lifestyle. Evidence-based practice depends on good research and good research depends on having a valid and reliable way to measure student achievement.

Valid outcome measures enable us to answer the following questions:
- What curricula are more effective and under what conditions for what outcomes?
- How do the standards relate to each other? For example, what is the relationship of skill in movement forms to participation in physical activity and fitness levels?

- How do we effectively instruct students to achieve the outcomes we target?
- How are good physical education programs related to academic achievement?

All of these questions are highly dependent upon having good measures of student performance. The NASPE assessment materials provide a foundation for measurement, data collection over time, and accountability by all.

Misuse of Assessment

Although assessment is a powerful tool to improve instruction and learning, there is the potential for unintended and negative consequences. When students are assessed on concepts and skills they have not been taught or have not been given sufficient time to learn, then assessment is not being used appropriately. When what is assessed becomes the whole curriculum rather than a measured sample of what students should be learning as a part of a comprehensive curriculum, assessment is being misused. When scores students receive on assessments are used exclusively to evaluate students, teachers, schools, districts, or states then assessment is being misused. While the NASPE assessments target critical outcomes that all students should achieve, they are not the only important outcomes of a good program.

In summary, assessments should be used to provide teachers, students, parents, administrators and policy makers with both formative and summative data. This information helps teachers improve instruction and demonstrate student learning. Administrators and policy makers may also use the data to determine the impact of physical education programs and support these programs.

National Association for Sport and Physical Education, an association of the American Alliance for Health, Physical Education, Recreation and Dance

11

National Association for Sport and Physical Education, an association of the American Alliance for Health, Physical Education, Recreation and Dance

Protocols Used to Administer and Code the NASPE Assessments

As part of the research protocol for this project, data was collected and coded according to a rubric connected to each assessment. All student performances were video recorded to facilitate analysis of data which included intra- and inter-rater reliability coding for data collection. Thousands of students participated in the national sample and provided data. The results of the coding enabled the task force to improve the quality and clarity of individual assessments and determine the most effective testing protocols.

For teachers using the NASPE assessments, video recording allows them to view a student's performance on more than one occasion. It enables greater scoring accuracy because the teacher can conduct an "instant replay" of an assessment by simply rewinding all or part of the record. Video recording also provides the teacher with hard evidence that can be used to document student achievement. Finally, video records provide a mechanism for the teacher to conduct periodic self-checks of his/her scoring reliability.

The next section of this manual contains protocols and directions for administering the assessments. The protocols and directions guide standardized administration of the assessments. If you are conducting summative assessments, the protocols must be followed precisely in order to later compare performances, pre and post, class to class, year to year, teacher to teacher or school to school. Before using the assessments (with the exception of pre-assessment), make sure students have been taught the task and have had numerous opportunities to practice the skills exactly as they are described in the assessment. Remember: be sure to follow school or district guidelines regarding permission to record student performances.

Protocols for Administering the Assessments and Collecting Data

Administering the Assessments

Preparation
1. Prepare the score sheets ahead of time and have pencils, clipboard, stopwatch and other activity equipment required for the assessment on site.
2. Prepare all equipment (and perhaps some spare equipment) before the class enters the assessment setting. This includes taping mats, inflating balls, distributing safety mats and removing objects/equipment around the perimeter of the space.
3. Prepare numbers and have safety pins or numbered pinnies/vests available prior to class. Make numbers as large as possible (10 inches high is suggested) in a color that contrasts with the shirt or pinnie/vest.
4. Assign numbers to students before class begins. Once students enter class, attach them to the front and/or back of the student depending on the assessment. Students must be easily identified by number throughout the entire assessment.
5. Do not give two students in one class the same number. If recording on multiple days or for multiple assessments, students should keep their same number. If a student is absent, do not reassign that number.
6. When there is an assessment with an offense and defense situation in the assessment, provide students a different color of pinnie/vest for offense and a different color of pinnie/vest for defense.

7. Prepare alternative activities for students who are not involved in the assessments. Ensure that these students are active, supervised, and safe.

8. Once the testing area is identified and marked, set up the camera and record a trial run of the assessment before class to be sure the viewfinder can "see" all essential elements of the entire assessment.

Video recording

1. When movement in rhythm to an accompaniment is part of the assessment, place camera and music source (if used) close together so the music can be heard when later reviewing the video record.

2. Camera setup directions for each assessment are provided in the individual assessments. Follow these for each assessment unless your testing situation requires a different set up. Ultimately, you must be able to see the entire activity area needed for an assessment, the trajectory or path of the ball or implement, the target when indicated, and the student's entire body (feet, head, student number). This may require moving some cameras further back if they do not have a wide-angle lens. It may also require adjusting the angle for the situation.

Safety considerations

1. The court or floor surface should be dry, clean, and clear of obstacles surrounding and beyond the boundary of the test area. Adequate out of bounds space is important for deceleration, turning and such.

2. If testing outdoors, the surface must be appropriate. A hard surface should be dry, smooth and clean. If the assessment calls for a grassy area, it should be appropriately mowed and free of grass clippings, hazards, trash, holes and obstructions.

3. Only safe footwear should be allowed; no sandals, boots, bare feet and such.

4. Be sure students know the boundaries of the testing area, understand the markings, are aware of the deceleration or stopping zone, and are very clear about where their personal space is located.

5. Set up the testing area so it cannot inadvertently be entered by other students.

6. During testing, have the student performing the assessment face away from distractions.

7. Have students empty their pockets, remove jewelry, tie their shoes and take off accessories that might injure them or a partner. This is especially important for assessments that require rolling or inverted positions and/or performance with or against another person.

Warm up and practice

1. A warm-up and short practice period is recommended. The assessments should not be a secret and students should have had adequate learning time in previous lessons.

2. Some assessments require students to perform routines that have been previously created and written down. Provide time for students to read and practice their previously created routines. Do not allow students to read the routines during the assessment. Do not read the routine to the students. Do not say the directions to a dance out loud during the assessment and do not use music that has the directions on the CD/tape.

Test administration

1. As noted above, camera setup directions for each activity are specifically described. Follow the directions for each assessment.

2. If possible, have a teacher administer the assessment and have another person video record the performance.

3. The teacher should read, "Directions to Students" exactly as they are written so that the directions are audible to the students and on the video recording.

4. Be sure all students understand the directions. Directions should be read to small groups of students immediately prior to assessments for kindergarten and 2nd grade and to the entire class for 5th graders. In this latter instance, teachers may need to periodically reread the instructions if a long period of time has elapsed since the instructions were initially read. Be fair. If it makes sense to read the instructions again for a student, do so.

5. Do not permit other students to act as an audience for those being assessed; make arrangements for others to be physically active and adequately supervised.

6. The order of the students on the code sheet should be the same as the order of the students on the video record. Student name and number as seen on the video should be recorded on the code sheet.

7. If feasible, each student should say his/her number in front of the camera in a loud voice immediately before attempting the assessment. Ask the student to stand 5 feet (sufficient distance to see number and body of student) in front of the camera and state his/her name and number clearly. Alternatively, the assistant doing the video recording could say the name and number of the students who are being assessed.

8. Use a "ready", "start" signal to begin the assessment.

9. When an assessment requires using first one foot and then the other, or move to the left and then right, or an out and return, instruct student to wait until you give him the signal to begin the second half of the assessment, the return, or the change of feet/hand. There should be a pause until "start" is indicated.

10. Be sure students know what to do if action is stopped, whether they can restart and what to do if the ball goes far out of bounds. Be sure students understand the important elements of an assessment (e.g., they may erroneously think speed is the critical element when in fact the critical elements are accurate passes and controlling receptions). Be sure students understand the difference between a jog and a walk. Be sure students understand that they should resume an interrupted skill during a timed assessment. Be sure students know that trials that don't make it past a certain line or height will not count in the total but that they can keep going and try to resume the correct distance/height until time is up.

Coding protocols

Study the assessment
1. Read the entire assessment carefully.
2. Study the major focus of each criterion.
3. Study the value difference of each level for all criteria, noting that level 3 equals competence.

Preview—View the video record before attempting to score
1. Look for the major focus of each criterion (practice for recognition of each).
2. Look for the differences in performance in relation to the quality level of each criterion (range of proficiency among performers; common errors).
3. Become familiar with the requirements of the criteria and corresponding performance levels of the assessments.

National Association for Sport and Physical Education, an association of the American Alliance for Health, Physical Education, Recreation and Dance

15

4. Some Level 4 criteria use the term, "fluid motion." This term was consciously chosen to separate Level 4 performers from Level 3 by emphasizing the flowing, smooth, and graceful nature of the performance. A Level 4 performance should be effortless, refined and performed without hesitation. Typically, only a very small number of students in each class will be able to demonstrate a Level 4 performance.

Practice scoring
1. View the first performer and make a decision about the first criterion and then all of the other criteria.
2. View as many times as necessary until a score can be determined consistently on each viewing.
3. If the performance includes multiple students (dance, game situations), focus on one student at a time, repeating the above steps for each.
4. Repeat until all students in the performance have been scored on all criteria.

Scoring (use score sheet designed for the specific assessment)
1. Record student number and gender.
2. Record scores for all criteria and trials and for all students as required by the assessment.
3. Total scores for all criteria and record on the score sheet in the designated column.
4. Repeat steps above for all performers on the video record.

Scoring sheet information
1. Fill out all of the scoring sheet for future use.
2. The school name and location should be written on the cover of the videotape or CD *and* on the videotape or CD itself (to prevent confusion if the cover is misplaced from the videotape or CD).

Preliminary Data Analysis

More than 4000 students were assessed at over 90 schools across the country, making this project one of the largest and most comprehensive analyses of the current state of movement performance among elementary school students in physical education class. Data from the assessments are being used in a multitude of ways: to inform teachers and guide curriculum, to motivate students, to inform parents, administrators and policy makers on student progress and to assist researchers.

Preliminary analyses of the pilot and national samples included extensive traditional test construction methodology, such as item difficulty ratings and discrimination indices which established evidence of validity. In addition, descriptive and inferential statistics of the pilot study samples (including age, gender, grade) were performed. A more contemporary analysis using item response theory (IRT) was also applied in order to establish validity.

This cutting edge approach examined item difficulty and discrimination for the purpose of equating assessments across grades and within grade levels. Equating allows teachers to compare students of different grades on different assessments. For example, 2nd graders jumping can be compared with 5th graders in-line skating to tell if the program shows progressive learning. Model data fit and categorization statistics were also established to make sure statistically that the data is really representative of the entire population.

Based on the analyses conducted, teachers should be confident that the NASPE assessments provide a clear and meaningful set of attainable expectations for students. The format and descriptive information in the rubrics provide students and teachers with targets for improved performance. In addition, researchers benefit from data analyses which are far more thorough than traditional skills tests analysis. This project sought to address the needs of teachers and students who will be the end-users of the assessments, as well as researchers who can use this as an example of new and dynamic measurement.

The overall results for this project are still being processed as data is collected. Current analyses show the assessments have appropriate difficulty and discriminate well among performance levels according to categorization statistics. Expected group differences are also well documented. The assessments have met the initial criteria; they are informative for teachers and students and have met further criteria, which is solid psychometric properties. It is the psychometric foundation of the assessments which distinguish this project from any other in the field. The assessments were developed by experts who have a strong theoretical and practical foundation in movement proficiency and the testing protocols and analyses were conducted by physical education measurement specialists.

Results from the final data analysis will be published in summer 2008 as an addendum to this publication and posted on the NASPE website at www.naspeinfo.org. The results will include descriptive data for each grade-level range and the validity and reliability estimates.

National Association for Sport and Physical Education, an association of the American Alliance for Health, Physical Education, Recreation and Dance

17

Table 1: Standard 1 Elementary Assessments

Kindergarten (N=8)	2nd grade (N=11)	5th grade (N=11)
Underhand Catching	Approach & Kick a Ball	Basketball: Dribble, Pass and Receive
Dribble with Hand	Dance Sequence	Basketball: Defense
Hopping	Dribble with Hand and Jog	Basketball: Offense
Running	Galloping	Dance
Sliding	Gymnastics Sequence	Floor Hockey: Dribble & Shoot
Striking	Jumping & Landing Combination	Gymnastics
Weight Transfer	Jump forward	Inline Skating
Underhand Throw	Locomotor Sequence	Overhand Throwing
	Overhand Catching	Soccer: Dribble, Pass, and Receive
	Skipping	Soccer: Offense
	Striking with Paddle	Striking with a Paddle

Physical Education Assessment Bank: Concept and Construction

In addition to the publication of the assessment materials, NASPE is developing a physical education assessment bank, which is a collection of assessments of a variety of tasks that share the same scale and are easily accessed for preparing task subsets tailored to a specific group (Umar, 1997). In other words, this bank will include assessments ranked for difficulty and allow a teacher to select appropriately difficult tasks for a student or class of students.

Construction of an assessment bank depends heavily on two major new advances in modern assessment practice; Item Response Theory (IRT) and test equating. IRT was developed during the 1950s and 60s in educational measurement practice. Its relatively slow development was accelerated in the 1980s by the growing accessibility of personal computers and development of application software. Today, IRT is the most dominant theory for test construction in all major testing organizations and agencies. When compared to measurement models based on the Classical Testing Theory (CTT), which has been the primary testing theory in the field of physical education, models based upon IRT have several advantages (Hambleton, Swaminathan, & Rogers, 1991; Spray, 1987). The primary advantages of IRT are that item parameters are independent of the ability level of the examinees responding to the items, and at the same time, the ability parameters are also independent of the items used in tests and the performance of other examinees. This is known as the "invariance" feature of IRT. Because of this feature, the interpretation of item difficulty and examinee ability is consistent in IRT. For example, a difficult item will not become easier when it is applied to a group of examinees with higher abilities. Another important advantage of IRT is that item difficulty and student ability are set on the same scale, which makes it much easier to determine the appropriateness of an item for a given ability level and to interpret test scores. As a result, a teacher can select an assessment that is appropriately difficult for a student and can explain what the student's score really means. IRT has been used in physical education for many years and has been well tested for its measurement advantages (see Spray, 1987, Safrit, Zhu, Costa, & Zhang, 1992; Zhu, 1996, 2006; Zhu & Cole, 1996; Zhu & Safrit, 1993, for more information).

Test equating is a statistical procedure used to establish the relationship between scores from two or more tests or to place them on a common scale. The task of equating, in general, is to establish statistically a conversion relationship among summary scores from two or more test forms or tests. The relationship could be linear or non-linear depending on the equating method employed. Test equating methods, according to the test theory on which they are based, generally can be classified into two categories: traditional and IRT (Kolen & Brennan, 2004; Zhu, 1998). With test equating, putting two or more tests on the same scale becomes possible, which is also necessary for establishing an item or assessment bank. A number of successful test equating applications in fitness testing based upon traditional equating approaches have been reported (Zhu, 1998, 2001). As a result, a teacher can select any one assessment and will be able to accurately anticipate a student's performance on a different and dissimilar assessment.

An assessment bank can provide several assessment advantages for teachers and data collectors. First, because the tasks are set on the same scale, testing scores generated will be equivalent to each other even when a different task is assessed. This allows cross-school comparison even when different tasks are used. In the past, cross-school comparisons were often established by using raw scores, rather than scaled scores. As a

National Association for Sport and Physical Education, an association of the American Alliance for Health, Physical Education, Recreation and Dance

19

result, the students' performances were often dependent on the difficulties of the assessments selected, making it very difficult to achieve objective cross-comparisons. With scaled scores, the difficulty of an assessment is taken into consideration for the scaling process. Therefore, students in first period class completing assessment X can be compared to students in second period who completed assessment Y.

Second, because the difficulty of each item in this set of assessments is known, and the discrimination ability between items is known, teachers can select assessment tasks which target specific levels of student learning. For example, a set of tasks is usually administered to all students; however, very difficult or easy items usually do not work well for students at low or high ends of the ability scale. These students either all score at the top (a level 4 performance), or all at the bottom (level 1). If that is the case, then the assessment has failed to discriminate and is generally ineffective at providing information about ability. With an assessment bank, assessments with appropriate difficulties for a targeted group can be selected. This selection process, known as computerized adaptive testing, can enable student assessment to be very time efficient. The teacher can select appropriately difficult assessments for each student, even though the assessments are different.

Third, development and application of new assessments becomes much easier with an assessment bank. In the past, when existing tests or items became too hard or too easy for a special population, separate tests were developed for that population, but scores from the newly developed tests could no longer be interpreted on the basis of the existing tests. The assessment bank concept can solve this problem. Instead of developing new tests, additional assessments targeted to the population to be tested can be developed and then linked to the existing bank. As a result, assessments sharing the same scale are accumulated and a complete bank can be formed gradually.

Finally, an assessment bank makes accurate assessing of student change/growth possible. Previously, when it became obvious that a task was either too hard or too easy for a student or groups of students, a different test was developed for them. The problem with that procedure was that the "new" test was not related to the original one, and there was no way to determine what a student's ability would be on the original test. With an assessment bank, this problem can be effectively eliminated because the scores will be equivalent even if they are generated from different tasks. Think of the process in this way: Suppose you wanted to determine a student's upper body strength and used a pull-up test as the assessment. There would have been a lot of "0" scores because the test was too difficult. Instead, a push-up assessment would yield far fewer "0" scores and the range of scores would be wider. Unless a link between the two assessments has been established, there would be no way to equate a score of 1 pull-up to a score of 5 push-ups. The process used in the NASPE assessment project allows teachers and researchers to equate different scores across students.

Conclusion

Physical fitness is not only one of the most important keys to a healthy body, it is the basis of dynamic and creative intellectual activity.

- John F. Kennedy

Assessing "classroom" subjects such as math and language arts is fairly straight-forward: subject matter is taught and homework, quizzes and written exams quantify student progress.

Physical education. a subject focused on physical competencies, is more complex. Nationally-recognized content standards did not exist until 1995 when the *National Standards for Physical Education* were published by NASPE. Since then, teachers have used various methods, or in some cases no method, to measure student progress and achievement of the standards. Establishing national standards was the first step in bringing physical education to a higher level of accountability. Establishing assessment guidelines, fully illustrated in *PE Metrics: Assessing the National Standards* is the second and final step in this process.

PE Metrics: Assessing the National Standards allows physical educators to confidently measure student success and accountability. Good health includes regular participation in physical activity, which starts with being a physically educated person. The time has never been better for properly educating and assessing our students in physical education.

National Association for Sport and Physical Education, an association of the American Alliance for Health, Physical Education, Recreation and Dance

21

National Association for Sport and Physical Education, an association of the American Alliance for Health, Physical Education, Recreation and Dance

Standard 1:

Demonstrates competency in motor skills and movement patterns needed to perform a variety of physical activities

Performance Indicator:

Throw, catch, dribble, kick, and strike from a stationary position

Assessment Task:

Continuously dribble a ball for 15 seconds with one hand

Criteria for Competence (Level 3):

1. Dribbles with all the selected essential elements:

   a) one hand contact

   b) maintains constant height of rebound

   c) pushes ball (no slapping)

2. Maintains a continuous dribble with feet staying within boundaries

■ Assessment Rubric:

Level	1. Form	2. Continuous Action & Control
4	Dribbles with all the selected essential elements with fluid motion	Maintains a continuous dribble with very little travel from the starting position for 15 seconds
3	Dribbles with all the selected essential elements: a) one hand contact b) maintains constant height of rebound c) pushes ball (no slapping)	Maintains a continuous dribble with feet staying within boundaries
2	Dribbles with 2 of 3 essential elements present	1 break in continuous dribble or moves outside of boundaries on one occasion
1	Dribbles with 1 or no essential elements present	Has more than 1 break in continuous dribble and/or moves outside of boundaries on more than one occasion
0	Violates safety procedures and/or does not complete the assessment task	

National Association for Sport and Physical Education, an association of the American Alliance for Health, Physical Education, Recreation and Dance

23

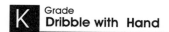
■ **Assessment Protocols:**

Directions for Students (Read aloud verbatim):

- Today I am going to watch you dribble.
- On my signal, start dribbling the ball using one hand, keeping the ball bouncing at the same height, pushing the ball without slapping it.
- Stay in your own square.
- Continue dribbling until I give the stop signal.

Directions for Teachers:

Preparation:

- See the manual for General Protocols for instruction, warm-up, camera location, and operation.
- Three students can be assessed at one time.
- Clearly indicate each student's personal space (3-foot square).
- Use your own start/stop signal allowing students to dribble for 15 seconds.
- The assessment is 1 trial (15 seconds).

Safety:

- Be sure students understand where their own square is located.
- If outside, use smooth hard surface that is free of obstructions.

Equipment/Materials:

- 3 properly inflated 10" playground balls
- Taped 3-foot squares on floor to designate personal space
- Stopwatch or clock for timing 15 seconds

Diagram of Space/Distances:

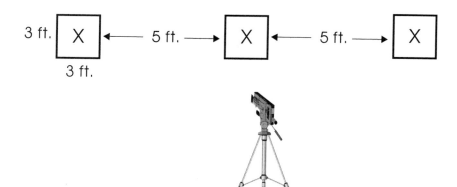

Camera Location and Operation:

Set up camera in front of the middle student and far enough away so that all 3 students can be viewed. The student's entire body, including the feet, must be in view and close enough to assess the form.

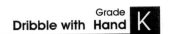
Assessment Score Sheet

PE Teacher _____   Grade _____   Date _____

School _____   Classroom Teacher _____

Student Name	ID Number	Gender	Form (0-4)	Continuous Action & Control (0-4)	Total Score (0-8) 6=Competent

K Grade
Hopping

Standard 1:

Demonstrates competency in motor skills and movement patterns needed to perform a variety of physical activities

Performance Indicator:

Demonstrate hopping, jumping, galloping, and sliding

Assessment Task:

Hop in place

Criteria for Competence (Level 3):

1. Hops, taking off from one foot and landing on the same foot. Performs action on other foot
2. Hops within self-space continuously for 10 seconds with no loss of balance or extraneous arm motion. Performs action on other foot

■ Assessment Rubric:

Level	1. Form*	2. Consistency of Action
4	Hops, taking off from one foot and landing on the same foot with smooth, balanced action. Correctly performs action on other foot	Hops within self-space continuously for 10 seconds with fluid motion and consistency on each foot
3	Hops, taking off from one foot and landing on the same foot. Performs action on other foot	Hops within self-space continuously for 10 seconds with no loss of balance or extraneous arm motion. Performs action on other foot
2	Performs hopping action correctly for one but not the other foot	Hops continuously for 10 seconds with no loss of balance, but does not stay in self space
1	Performs hopping action incorrectly for both feet	Loses balance or cannot sustain hopping motion on both left and right foot for 10 seconds
0	Violates safety procedures and/or does not complete the assessment task	

*Example of incorrect hopping action includes: foot does not leave the floor, one foot to the other foot, and one foot to two feet.

■ Assessment Protocols:

Directions for Students (Read aloud verbatim):

- Today I am going to watch you hop.
- Stand in the middle of your own square.
- On my signal, start hopping on one foot in your square until I give the stop signal.
- Then I will ask you to switch to your other foot.
- I am looking to see if you take off and land on the same foot without stopping or moving outside your square for 10 seconds.

Directions for Teachers:

Preparation:

- See the manual for General Protocols for instruction, warm-up, camera location, and operation.
- Three students can be assessed at one time.
- Clearly indicate each student's personal square (3-foot square).
- Use your own start/stop signal allowing students to hop for 10 seconds on each foot.

Safety:

- Be sure students understand where their personal space is located.
- Allow only safe footwear (no sandals, boots, bare feet, etc.).
- If outside, use smooth hard surface that is free of obstructions.

Equipment/Materials:

- Taped 3-foot squares to designate personal space area
- Stopwatch or clock for timing 10 seconds

Diagram of Space/Distances:

Use taped 3-foot squares on the floor to designate personal space area for 3 students with 5 feet between each.

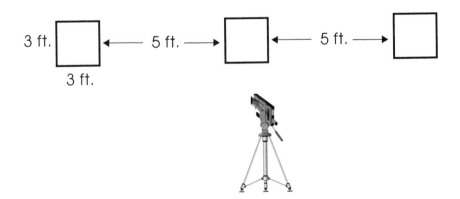

Camera Location and Operation:

Set up camera in front of the middle student and far enough away so that all 3 students can be viewed. The student's entire body, including the feet, must be in view and close enough to assess the form.

National Association for Sport and Physical Education, an association of the American Alliance for Health, Physical Education, Recreation and Dance

27

Assessment Score Sheet

PE Teacher _____ Grade _____ Date _____

School _____ Classroom Teacher _____

Student Name	ID Number	Gender	Form (0-4)	Consistency of Action (0-4)	Total Score (0-8) 6=Competent

National Association for Sport and Physical Education, an association of the American Alliance for Health, Physical Education, Recreation and Dance

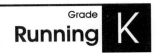
Standard 1:

Demonstrates competency in motor skills and movement patterns needed to perform a variety of physical activities

Performance Indicator:

Demonstrate a mature pattern of running

Assessment Task:

Run continuously for 60 feet

Criteria for Competence (Level 3):

1. Runs with the essential elements of a mature pattern:

   a) arm/leg opposition

   b) toes point forward

   c) arms swing forward/backward and do not cross midline of body

   d) feet land heel to toe

2. Runs in straight pathway without stumbling, stopping or falling down

■ Assessment Rubric:

Level	1. Form	2. Consistency of Action
4	Displays all the essential elements of a mature pattern with fluid motion	Runs smoothly in straight pathway without breaks in stride
3	Runs with the essential elements of a mature pattern: a) Arm /leg opposition b) Toes point forward c) Arms swing forward/backward and do not cross midline of body d) Feet land heel to toe	Runs in straight pathway without stumbling, stopping, or falling down
2	Runs with 3 of 4 essential elements present	Runs without stopping or falling down, but stumbles, runs in erratic pathway, or has inconsistent stride
1	Runs with 2 or fewer essential elements present	Stops running action or falls down
0	Violates safety procedures and/or does not complete the assessment task	

National Association for Sport and Physical Education, an association of the American Alliance for Health, Physical Education, Recreation and Dance

29

■ **Assessment Protocols:**

Directions for Students (Read aloud verbatim):

- Today I am going to watch you run.
- Stand behind the starting line.
- On my signal, run fast all the way through the course.
- Stay in the running lane by running in a straight line.
- Do not stop running until after you cross the finish line.
- Run as fast as you can showing me your best running form by swinging your arms forward and backward, having your toes pointed forward, and landing on the heel of your foot first.

Directions for Teachers:

Preparation:

- See the manual for General Protocols for instruction, warm-up, camera location, and operation.
- The assessment can be set up inside or outside.
- Clearly indicate the running lane area and finish line.
- Emphasize to students that they should not stop running until **after** they cross the finish line.

Safety:

- Be sure students understand where the finish line is located.
- Allow only safe footwear (no sandals, boots, bare feet, etc.).
- If outside, use smooth safe surface that is free of obstructions.

Equipment/Materials:

- 4 cones to mark the starting line and finish line

Diagram of Space/Distances:

Use cones to form a lane 5 feet wide and 60 feet long with an additional 15 feet of unobstructed space beyond the finish line (total of 75 feet long). Start line is at least 3 feet from any obstruction and finish line at least 15 feet from any obstruction.

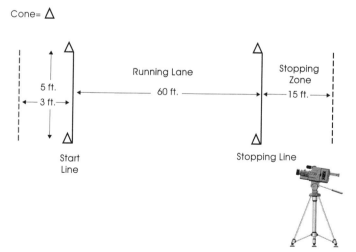

Camera Location and Operation:

Set up camera near end of running lane but outside cones, so that student can be viewed running toward the finish line. The student's entire body, including the feet, must be in view and close enough to assess the form. Be sure that you can view student's form from start to finish.

Assessment Score Sheet

PE Teacher _____   Grade _____   Date _____

School _____   Classroom Teacher _____

Student Name	ID Number	Gender	Form (0-4)	Consistency of Action (0-4)	Total Score (0-8) 6=Competent

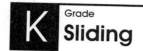

Grade K
Sliding

Standard 1:

Demonstrates competency in motor skills and movement patterns needed to perform a variety of physical activities

Performance Indicator:

Demonstrate hopping, jumping, galloping, and sliding

Assessment Task:

Slide continuously for 30 feet with the preferred foot leading

Criteria for Competence (Level 3):

1. Slides with selected essential elements:
   a) uses a step-close action
   b) maintains a side orientation without twisting hips (lead foot may turn out slightly in the direction of the slide)
   c) same foot leading
   d) brief period of non-support
2. Slides without losing continuity of the action

■ Assessment Rubric:

Level	1. Form	2. Consistency of Action
4	Displays all the selected essential elements with fluid motion	Slides smoothly without losing continuity of the action
3	Slides with selected essential elements: a) uses a step-close action b) maintains a side orientation without twisting hips (lead foot may turn out slightly) c) same foot leading d) brief period of non-support	Slides without losing continuity of the action
2	Slides with 3 of 4 essential elements	Loses the continuity of the action
1	Slides with 2 or fewer essential elements	Stops sliding action or falls down
0	Violates safety procedures and/or does not complete the assessment task	

National Association for Sport and Physical Education, an association of the American Alliance for Health, Physical Education, Recreation and Dance

NASPE

■ **Assessment Protocols:**

Directions for Students (Read aloud verbatim):

- Today I am going to watch you slide.
- Stand with your side to the starting line.
- On my signal, slide to the end of the lane, without stopping, and cross the finish line.
- Stay in the lane.
- This is not a race.
- Show me your best sliding form by
  a) using a step/close pattern with the same foot leading;
  b) moving sideways without twisting your hips.

Directions for Teachers:

Preparation:

- See the manual for General Protocols for instruction, warm-up, camera location, and operation.
- Clearly indicate the lane area and start and finish lines.

Safety:

- Be sure students understand where the end lines are located.
- Allow only safe footwear (no sandals, boots, bare feet, etc.).
- If outside, use smooth hard surface that is free of obstructions.

Equipment/Materials:

- 4 cones and floor tape to mark the starting line and finish line

Diagram of Space/Distances:

Use cones to form a lane 5 feet wide and 30 feet long with an additional 15 feet of unobstructed space beyond the finish line (total of 45 feet long). Starting line is at least 3 feet from any obstruction and finish line at least 15 feet from any obstruction.

Cone= △

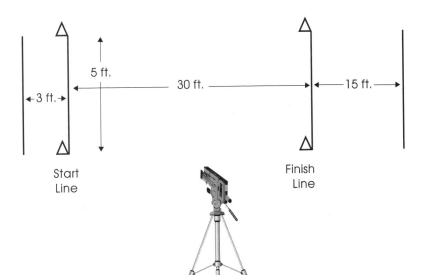

Camera Location and Operation:

Set up camera at middle of lane outside cones so that student (and the start and finish line) can be viewed for the entire sliding motion while facing the camera. The student's entire body, including the feet, must be in view and close enough to assess the form without moving the camera to follow the action.

National Association for Sport and Physical Education, an association of the American Alliance for Health, Physical Education, Recreation and Dance

33

Assessment Score Sheet

PE Teacher _____ Grade _____ Date _____

School _____ Classroom Teacher _____

Student Name	ID Number	Gender	Form (0-4)	Consistency of Action (0-4)	Total Score (0-8) 6=Competent

National Association for Sport and Physical Education, an association of the American Alliance for Health, Physical Education, Recreation and Dance

Standard 1:

Demonstrates competency in motor skills and movement patterns needed to perform a variety of physical activities

Performance Indicator:

Throw, catch, dribble, kick, and strike from a stationary position

Assessment Task:

Continuously strike a balloon with a short-handled paddle using an underhand pattern for 20 seconds

Criteria for Competence (Level 3):

1. Displays all of the selected essential elements with no more than 2 errors in form during the entire assessment:
   a) visual tracking
   b) flat paddle surface
   c) upward underhand striking pattern using one hand
2. Displays all of the essential elements:
   a) consistently sends the balloon higher than the head
   b) stays within the boundaries
   c) maintains continuous striking action

■ Assessment Rubric:

Level	1. Form	2. Continuous Strikes & Boundaries
4	Displays all the selected essential elements with fluid motion without error	Always sends the balloon higher than the head Maintains continous striking action Very little travel from the starting position
3	Displays all the selected essential elements with no more that 2 errors in form during the entire assessment: a) visual tracking b) flat paddle surface c) upward underhand striking pattern using one hand	Displays all of the essential elements: a) consistently sends the balloon higher than the head b) stays within the boundaries c) maintains continuous striking action
2	Displays all the selected essential elements with no more than 3 errors in form during the entire assessment	Strikes with 2 of the 3 essential elements present
1	Displays all the selected essential elements with 4 or more errors in form during the entire assessment	Strikes with 1 or no essential elements present
0	Violates safety procedures and/or does not complete the assessment task	

Consistently = above 90%   Usually = 75% - 89%   Sometimes = 50% -74%   Seldom = below 50%

National Association for Sport and Physical Education, an association of the American Alliance for Health, Physical Education, Recreation and Dance

35

■ **Assessment Protocols:**

Directions for Students (Read aloud verbatim):

- Today I am going to watch you strike a balloon with a paddle.
- I am looking to see if you keep the paddle flat, watch the balloon, and use a one-handed underhand motion.
- Strike the balloon at your waist, but make it go higher than your head.
- Keep the balloon in the air.
- You should stay within your personal square. If you go outside your space, continue striking and try to move back into the square.
- Keep striking the balloon until I say stop. If the balloon falls to the floor, pick it up and resume.

Directions for Teachers:

Preparation:

- See the manual for General Protocols for instruction, warm-up, camera location, and operation.
- Clearly indicate the personal space area.
- The assessment is 20 seconds.

Safety:

- Be sure students understand where their personal space is located.
- If outside, use smooth hard surface that is free of obstructions.

Equipment/Materials:

- 1 short-handled foam, wooden, or plastic paddle
- 1 balloon per student (round balloons fully inflated)
- Floor tape
- Stopwatch or clock for timing.

Diagram of space/Distances:

Create a 10 ft. by 10 ft. square with floor tape to designate personal space area.

S=student

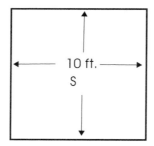

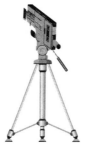

Camera Location and Operation:

Set up camera in front of the student and far enough away so that the entire personal space area can be viewed. The student's entire body, including the feet, must be in view and close enough to assess the form.

Assessment Score Sheet

PE Teacher _____   Grade _____   Date _____

School _____   Classroom Teacher _____

Student Name	ID Number	Gender	Form (0-4)	Continuous Strikes & Boundaries (0-4)	Total Score (0-8) 6=Competent

National Association for Sport and Physical Education, an association of the American Alliance for Health, Physical Education, Recreation and Dance

37

K Grade Underhand Catching

Standard 1:

Demonstrates competency in motor skills and movement patterns needed to perform a variety of physical activities

Performance Indicator:

Throw, catch, dribble, kick, and strike from a stationary position

Assessment Task:

Catch a ball tossed by a teacher using an underhand catching pattern

Criteria for Competence: (Level 3)

1. Attempts the catch with selected essential elements:

   a) hands reach to meet the ball

   b) uses hands without trapping ball against chest

   c) does not turn head away from ball

2. Successfully catches the ball

■ Assessment Rubric:

Level	1. Form	2. Catching Success
4	Displays all the selected essential elements with fluid motion	Catches the ball with no bobbles
3	Attempts the catch with selected essential elements: a) hands reach to meet ball b) uses hands without trapping ball against chest c) does not turn head away from ball	Successfully catches the ball
2	Attempts to catch with 2 of 3 essential elements present	Catches the ball but then fumbles and recovers it
1	Attempts to catch with 1 or no essential elements	Catches the ball then drops it or fails to catch the ball
0	Violates safety procedures and/or does not complete the assessment task	

National Association for Sport and Physical Education, an association of the American Alliance for Health, Physical Education, Recreation and Dance

■ Assessment Protocols:

Directions for Students (Read aloud verbatim):

- Today I am going to watch you catch.
- Get ready to catch the ball that I am throwing underhand to you.
- You don't have to stay on the starting spot. You may move to catch the ball.
- Show me your best catching form—hands ready, reach for the ball and catch the ball with your hands.
- You will get 3 chances to catch the ball.

Directions for Teachers:

- See the manual for General Protocols for instruction, warm-up, camera location, and operation.
- Clearly indicate where student should stand (6' from teacher).
- Toss ball gently using underhand action so ball drops toward student's waist.
- If it is a poor toss you may repeat the toss. Please indicate verbally on the tape that the toss will be repeated.
  Note: Ball may touch chest after it has been stopped and controlled with the hands.
- Remind student that they may move from the starting spot to catch the ball.
- Score each trial separately.

Safety:

Set up catching area so that no other students can enter it.

Equipment/Materials:

- 1- 8" playground ball
- 2 spots or lines marked on floor

Diagram of Space/Distance:

S=Student
T=Teacher

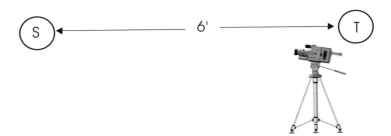

Camera Location and Operation:

Set up camera beside the teacher so that it points directly toward the student. The student's entire body, including the feet, must be in view and close enough to assess the form.

National Association for Sport and Physical Education, an association of the American Alliance for Health, Physical Education, Recreation and Dance

39

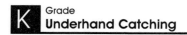
Assessment Score Sheet

PE Teacher _____   Grade _____   Date _____

School _____   Classroom Teacher _____

Student Name	ID Number	Gender	Form- 3 Trials (0-4)			Catching Success 3 Trials (0-4)			Total Score (0-24) 18=Competent
			1st	2nd	3rd	1st	2nd	3rd	

National Association for Sport and Physical Education, an association of the American Alliance for Health, Physical Education, Recreation and Dance

Standard 1:

Demonstrates competency in motor skills and movement patterns needed to perform a variety of physical activities

Performance Indicator:

Throw, catch, dribble, kick, and strike from a stationary position

Assessment Task:

Use an underhand throwing pattern to send a ball forward through the air to a large target

Criteria for Competence (Level 3):

1. Throws with selected essential elements:
   a) arm back in preparation
   b) opposite foot forward
   c) release of ball in forward direction
2. Hits target area on wall

■ Assessment Rubric:

Level	1. Form	2. Distance & Boundaries
4	Displays all the selected essential elements with fluid motion	Hits target area on wall with force
3	Throws with selected essential elements: a) arm back in preparation b) opposite foot forward c) release of ball in forward direction	Hits target area on wall
2	Throws with 2 of 3 essential elements present	Ball airborne for at least 10 feet but does not hit target
1	Throws with only 1 essential element present	Ball is airborne less than 10 feet
0	Violates safety procedures and/or does not complete the assessment task	

Note: Failure to use underhand throwing pattern (e.g., sidearm or overhand) is Incomplete Assessment Task (0).

National Association for Sport and Physical Education, an association of the American Alliance for Health, Physical Education, Recreation and Dance

41

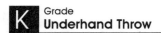

■ **Assessment Protocols:**

Directions for Students (Read aloud verbatim):

- Today I am going to watch you throw underhand.
- Stand behind the throwing line.
- Do not put your fingers in the holes in the ball.
- On my signal, throw the ball underhand and try to hit the large square on the wall.
- Show me your best throwing form by getting your arm back, stepping with the foot that's on the other side of the arm you are throwing with, and letting go of the ball in a forward direction.
- You will have 3 trials.

Directions for Teachers:

Preparation:

- See the manual for General Protocols for instruction, warm-up, camera location, and operation.
- Clearly indicate the throwing lane on the floor.
- The assessment is 3 trials.
- Be sure students do not put their fingers in the whiffle ball holes.
- If assessment is taking place outdoors, it should not be on a windy day.

Safety:

- Set up throwing area so that no other students can enter it.

Equipment/Materials:

- 4 whiffle balls (softball sized)
- Tape to form throwing line (6-foot line, and target square)
- 4 cones to form throwing lane and the airborne line

Diagram of Space/Distances:

Use tape to mark a throwing line on the floor 15 feet from a wall. Place another line on the floor 10 feet from the throwing line to mark minimal airborne distance. Mark a 10 foot by 10 foot target square on the wall. Place the target square 3 ' off the floor. Place a cone at each end of each line.

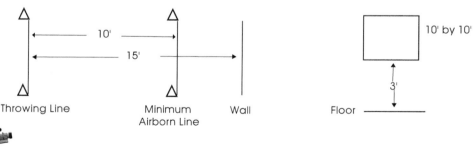

Camera Location and Operation:

Set up camera on an angle so that the student and the wall are visible. The student's entire body, including the feet, must be in view and close enough to assess the form.

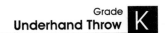
Assessment Score Sheet

PE Teacher _____   Grade _____   Date _____

School _____   Classroom Teacher _____

Student Name	ID Number	Gender	Form (0-4) Trials			Distance & Boundaries (0-4) Trials			Total Score (0-24) 18=Competent
			1st	2nd	3rd	1st	2nd	3rd	

National Association for Sport and Physical Education, an association of the American Alliance for Health, Physical Education, Recreation and Dance

43

K Grade
Weight Transfer

Standard 1:

Demonstrates competency in motor skills and movement patterns needed to perform a variety of physical activities

Performance Indicator:

Transfer weight hands/feet

Assessment Task:

Place weight on the hands and transfer feet sideways over a raised bar and back to the starting position

Criteria for Competence (Level 3):

1. Transfers weight to hands with selected essential elements:

   a) simultaneously taking off on 2 feet

   b) simultaneously landing on 2 feet

   c) hands maintaining stationary contact with the floor

2. Transfers weight momentarily to hands only without contacting the bar or falling down

■ Assessment Rubric:

Level	1. Form	2. Weight Support & Control
4	Displays all the selected essential elements with fluid motion	Transfers weight from feet to hands to feet with smooth action
3	Transfers weight to hands with selected essential elements: a) simultaneously taking off on 2 feet b) simultaneously landing on 2 feet c) hands maintaining stationary contact with the floor	Transfers weight to hands without feet contacting the bar or falling down
2	Transfers weight with 2 of 3 essential elements present	Transfers weight to hands without falling down but feet contact the bar
1	Transfers weight with only 1 essential element present	Feet fail to cross bar or student falls down
0	Violates safety procedures and/or does not complete the assessment task	

National Association for Sport and Physical Education, an association of the American Alliance for Health, Physical Education, Recreation and Dance

NASPE

■ **Assessment Protocols:**

Directions for Students (Read aloud verbatim):

- Today I am going to watch you put your weight on your hands.
- Stand on your personal space marker.
- On my signal, place both hands on the floor, <u>one hand on each side of the line</u>, keeping your feet on the marker.
- On my signal, "Over," take off from two feet shifting all of your weight onto your hands, cross the bar, without your feet touching it, and land on the other side with two feet.
- Your hands should stay on the floor.
- Then jump your feet back over the line to your marker, two feet taking off, two feet landing, at the same time, then stand up.
- You will do this two times.
- Ready? Over, back, STAND. Wait.
- Ready? Over, back STAND.

Directions for Teachers:

Preparation:

- See the manual for General Protocols for instruction, warm-up, camera location, and operation.
- Place a line 6' long on the floor. On the back half of the line, place a raised bar 3 feet long and 6" high. You might use a yardstick supported by two 6" cones. Mark where hands should be placed and mark where feet should be placed in starting position. See diagram.
- Make three stations five feet apart. Three students can be assessed at one time.
- Clearly indicate each student's personal marker where feet should be positioned to begin.
- Have students stand on their markers beside the bar so all are facing the same direction.
- Be sure to use the commands, "over, back, STAND" for each trial.
- The assessment consists of 2 trials.

Safety:

- Tape bar to supports (e.g., cones) so that it does not fall off if students hit the bar with their feet.
- If outside, use smooth surface that is free of obstructions.

Equipment/Materials:

- Tape for indicating hand and foot markers, lines, and holding bar in place
- 3 yardsticks (bars)
- Six 6-inch cones

National Association for Sport and Physical Education, an association of the American Alliance for Health, Physical Education, Recreation and Dance

45

Diagram of Space/Distances:

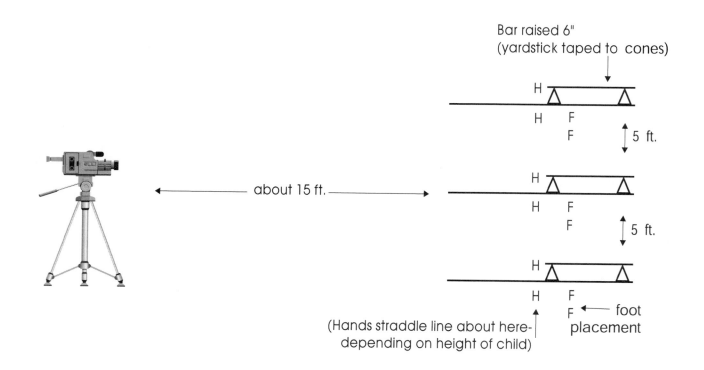

Bar raised 6"
(yardstick taped to cones)

about 15 ft.

5 ft.

5 ft.

H H F F
H H F F
H H F F

foot placement

(Hands straddle line about here-
depending on height of child)

Camera Location and Operation:

Set up camera in front of the middle student and far enough away <u>so that all 3 students can be viewed</u>. The student's entire body, including the feet, must be in view and close enough to assess the form.

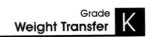

Assessment Score Sheet

PE Teacher _____   Grade _____   Date _____

School _____   Classroom Teacher _____

Student Name	ID Number	Gender	Form (0-4) Trials		Wt. Support & Control (0-4) Trials		Total Score (0-16) 12=Competent
			1st	2nd	1st	2nd	

National Association for Sport and Physical Education, an association of the American Alliance for Health, Physical Education, Recreation and Dance

47

Approach and Kick a Ball 2

Standard 1:

Demonstrates competency in motor skills and movement patterns needed to perform a variety of physical activities

Performance Indicator:

Dribble, kick, throw, catch, and strike a ball

Assessment Task:

Approach a stationary ball at a jog and kick with enough force to send it a distance of 30 feet on a smooth, level surface

Criteria for Competence (Level 3):

1. Kicks from a jog with selected essential elements:

   a) support foot to the side of the ball

   b) continuous motion into kick

   c) contact with instep (top of foot/shoelaces)

   d) follow through

2. Ball reaches target line between the cones

■ Assessment Rubric:

Level	1. Form	2. Distance and Accuracy
4	Displays all the selected essential elements with fluid motion	Ball reaches target line between the cones with good speed
3	Kicks from a jog with selected essential elements: a) support foot to the side of the ball b) continuous motion into kick c) contact with instep (top of foot/shoelaces) d) follow through	Ball reaches target line between the cones
2	Kicks from a jog with 3 of 4 essential elements present	Ball doesn't reach target line **or** is not between the cones
1	Kicks without jogging approach and 2 or fewer essential elements present	Ball does not reach the target line **and** is not between the cones
0	Violates safety procedures and/or does not complete the assessment task	

National Association for Sport and Physical Education, an association of the American Alliance for Health, Physical Education, Recreation and Dance

49

■ Assessment Protocols:

Directions for Students (Read aloud verbatim):

- Today I'm going to look at how you kick the ball from a jog.
- On my signal, jog to the ball and kick it without stopping. Kick it between the cones to the target line.
- Be sure to place your non-kicking foot to the side of the ball, prepare the kicking leg, contact the ball with the top of your foot or shoelaces, and follow through.
- You will kick 3 times.

Directions for Teachers:

Preparation:

- See the manual for General Protocols for instruction, warm-up, camera location, and operation.
- Clearly indicate the kicking lane on the floor.
- If assessment is conducted outside, use a hard surface, not grass.
- If keeping the ball stationary is a problem, place a small item under the ball (e.g., gauze, facial cleansing pad, or putty).

Safety:

- Set up kicking area so that no other students can enter it.

Equipment/Materials:

- 4 playground balls (12")
- Tape to form kicking line and target line on floor
- 8 cones to form kicking lane

Diagram of Space/Distances:

Use tape to form a kicking line and a target line (30' away) on the floor. Each line should be 8' long. Kicking line should be at least 10' from any obstruction (approach area). Place 4 cones 10' apart on each side of the kicking lane which is 8' wide.

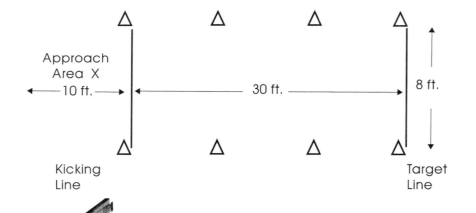

Camera Location and Operation:

Set up camera so that student's aproach, kicking lane, and target line can be viewed. The student's entire body, including the feet, must be in view and close enough to assess the form.

Assessment Score Sheet

PE Teacher _____   Grade _____   Date _____

School _____   Classroom Teacher _____

Student Name	ID Number	Gender	Form (0-4)			Distance & Accuracy (0-4)			Total Score (0-24) 18=Competent
			1st	2nd	3rd	1st	2nd	3rd	

National Association for Sport and Physical Education, an association of the American Alliance for Health, Physical Education, Recreation and Dance

51

2 | Grade
Dance Sequence

Standard 1:

Demonstrates competency in motor skills and movement patterns needed to perform a variety of physical activities

Performance Indicator:

Perform dance sequences to music

Assessment Task:

Perform to music a grade-level appropriate individual or partner dance that utilizes 3 different patterns

Criteria for Competency (Level 3):

1. Usually performs patterns and transitions correctly
2. Usually moves to the beat of the music

■ Assessment Rubric:

Level	1. Patterns & Transitions	2. Beat of the Music
4	Consistently performs patterns and transitions correctly	Consistently moves to the beat of the music
3	Usually performs patterns and transitions correctly	Usually moves to the beat of the music
2	Sometimes performs patterns and transitions correctly	Sometimes moves to the beat of the music
1	Seldom performs patterns and transitions correctly	Seldom moves to the beat of the music
0	Violates safety procedures and/or does not complete the assessment task	

Consistently = above 90%

Usually = 75% - 89%

Sometimes = 50% -74%

Seldom = below 50%

National Association for Sport and Physical Education, an association of the American Alliance for Health, Physical Education, Recreation and Dance

■ **Assessment Protocols:**

Directions for Students (Read aloud verbatim):

- Today I'm going to look at your dance sequence.
- When the music starts, begin the dance and continue until the music stops.
- Stay inside the square.
- Show me your best dance by performing each step correctly, with smooth transitions, and to the beat of the music.
- Don't stop until the music stops.

Directions for Teachers:

Preparation:

- See the manual for General Protocols for instruction, warm-up, camera location, and operation.
- Six students can be assessed at one time within a 20' x 20' square performance area.
- Repeat the dance as many times as necessary to assess all children.

Safety:

- Be sure students understand where to start and the boundaries of the performance area.
- Allow only safe footwear (no sandals, slides, boots, bare feet, etc.).
- If outside, use smooth hard surface that is free of obstructions.

Equipment/Materials:

- Use tape or 6-8 cones to form a 20' x 20' area
- Teacher-selected music for grade-level appropriate dance that utilizes 3 different step patterns
- CD/cassette player
- See Appendix for grade-level appropriate dances and resources

Diagram of Space/Distances:

△=Cone

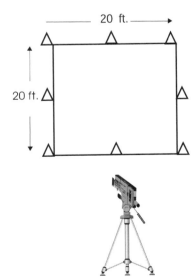

20 ft.

20 ft. △

Camera Location and Operation:

Set up camera outside cones so that entire performance area can be viewed. The students' entire bodies, including the feet, must be in view and close enough to assess the patterns.

National Association for Sport and Physical Education, an association of the American Alliance for Health, Physical Education, Recreation and Dance

53

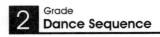

Assessment Score Sheet

PE Teacher _____   Grade _____   Date _____

School _____   Classroom Teacher _____

Student Name	ID Number	Gender	Patterns & Transitions (0-4)	Beat of the Music (0-4)	Total Score (0-8) 6=Competence

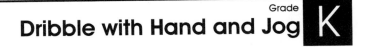

Grade

Dribble with Hand and Jog **K**

Standard 1:
Demonstrates competency in motor skills and movement patterns needed to perform a variety of physical activities

Performance Indicator:
Dribble, kick, throw, catch, and strike a ball

Assessment Task:
Dribble a ball with one hand to a cone and back while jogging slowly

Criteria for Competence (Level 3):
1. Dribbles with selected essential elements:
   a) pushing action of finger pads
   b) ball at approximately waist height
   c) ball in front of body and to the "dribble hand" side of the midline
2. Maintains a slow jog with some variation in speed while dribbling the designated distance
3. Maintains a continuous dribble within the boundaries

■ Assessment Rubric:

Level	1. Form	2. Space & Distance	3. Ball Control
4	Displays all the selected essential elements with fluid motion	Maintains consistent speed throughout the task	Maintains a smooth (no change in rhythm) continuous dribble within the boundaries
3	Dribbles with selected essential elements: a) pushing action of finger pads b) ball at approx. waist height c) ball in front of body and to the "dribble hand" side of the midline	Maintains a slow jog with some variation in speed while dribbling the designated distance	Maintains a continuous dribble within the boundaries
2	Dribbles with 2 of 3 essential elements present	Fails to maintain the jog or walks part of the designated distance	Stops dribbling <u>or</u> ball goes outside the boundaries
1	Dribbles with only 1 essential element present	Does not jog while dribbling the designated distance	Stops dribbling <u>and</u> ball goes outside the boundaries
0	Violates safety procedures and/or does not complete the assessment task		

Note: Control of ball and body is very important as children begin to travel at a rate higher than walking. The differences are often seen in walking versus jogging and being able to control ball and body to circle the cone and stop at finish/starting line.

National Association for Sport and Physical Education, an association of the American Alliance for Health, Physical Education, Recreation and Dance

55

■ **Assessment Protocols:**

Directions for Students (Read aloud verbatim):

- Today I'm going to look at how you dribble while jogging.
- Stand behind the starting line.
- On my signal, dribble the ball down to the large cone while you jog slowly and stay within your own lane.
- Dribble around the cone while jogging and back to the starting line.
- This is not a race.
- We are looking to see if you show good dribbling form by using your finger pads to push the ball, keeping the ball in front of you about waist height and keeping the ball to the front and "dribble hand" side of your body, while you maintain a slow jog with good control.
- Keep dribbling and jogging until you return to the starting line.

Directions for Teachers:

Preparation:

- See the manual for General Protocols for instruction, warm-up, camera location, and operation.
- Clearly indicate the starting/finish line, lane area and turning point.

Safety:

- Be sure students understand where the starting/finish line and turning cone are located.
- Allow only safe footwear (no sandals, slides, boots, bare feet, etc.).
- If outside, use smooth hard surface that is free of obstructions.

Equipment/Materials:

- 1 adequately inflated 10 or 12 inch playground ball
- 8 small cones to form lane
- 1 large cone to turn around
- Floor tape to form the starting/ finish line

Diagram of Space/Distances:

Use cones to form a lane 5 feet wide and 30 feet long with an additional 10 feet of unobstructed space behind the starting/finish line and 10 feet beyond the turning point (total of 50 feet). Cones should be placed down each lane line 10 ft apart to mark the lane lines. One large cone placed in middle of lane at 30' from starting/finish line will indicate the turn-around mark.

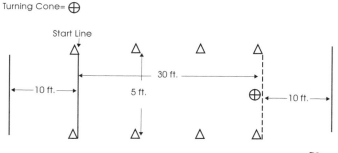

Camera Location and Operation:

Set up camera at turning zone but outside cones, so that student can be viewed dribbling into and making the turn. The student's entire body, including the feet, must be in view and close enough to assess the form.

56

National Association for Sport and Physical Education, an association of the American Alliance for Health, Physical Education, Recreation and Dance

Assessment Score Sheet

PE Teacher _____   Grade _____   Date _____

School _____   Classroom Teacher _____

Student Name	ID Number	Gender	Form (0-4)	Speed & Distance (0-4)	Control (0-4)	Total Score (0-12) 9=Competent

2 Grade
Galloping

Standard 1:

Demonstrates competency in motor skills and movement patterns needed to perform a variety of physical activities

Performance Indicator:

Demonstrates a mature pattern of jumping, galloping, sliding, and skipping

Assessment Task:

Gallop continuously for 30 feet with one foot leading. Repeat the task with the other foot leading

Criteria for Competence (Level 3):

1. Gallops with the essential elements of a mature pattern:
   a) same foot leading
   b) forward orientation
   c) moment of non-support
   d) back foot does not move in front of lead foot
2. Gallops with no break in action for 30', turns, and gallops back to the start with the other foot leading

■ Assessment Rubric:

Level	1. Form	2. Consistency
4	Displays all the essential elements of a mature pattern with fluid motion for entire task	Gallops smoothly with continuous action with each foot leading
3	Gallops with the essential elements of a mature pattern for entire task: a) same foot leading b) forward orientation c) moment of non-support d) back foot does not move in front of lead foot	Gallops with no break in action for 30', turns, and gallops back to the start with the other foot leading
2	Gallops with only 3 of 4 essential elements present	Gallops with no more than 1 break in action for entire task, turns, and gallops back to the start with other foot leading
1	Gallops with 2 or fewer essential elements present	Two or more breaks in action and/or does not return to the start with the other foot leading
0	Violates safety procedures and/or does not complete the assessment task	

National Association for Sport and Physical Education, an association of the American Alliance for Health, Physical Education, Recreation and Dance

■ Assessment Protocols:

Directions for Students (Read aloud verbatim):

- Today I'm going to look at your galloping.
- Stand behind the starting line.
- On my signal, gallop to the end of the lane with one foot leading.
- Stop, then turn around and gallop back with the other foot leading.
- Stay in your lane.
- This is not a race.
- Show me your best galloping form by using the same foot to lead, facing forward, bringing your feet together without crossing them and without stopping your movement.

Directions for Teachers:

Preparation:

- See the manual for General Protocols for instruction, warm-up, camera location, and operation.
- Clearly indicate the lane area and stopping zones.
- Remind students to switch lead feet once they reach the stopping line, for the return.
- Then same student turns around and gallops back with other foot leading.
- Do not designate right foot or left foot. Use terms "one foot" and "the other foot."

Safety:

- Be sure students understand where the start and end of the lane are located.
- Allow only safe footwear (no sandals, boots, bare feet, etc.).
- If outside, use smooth hard surface that is free of obstructions.

Equipment/Materials:

- At least 8 cones to form lane
- Floor tape to form starting line and finish line

Diagram of Space/Distances:

Use cones to form a lane 5 feet wide and 30 feet long with an additional 10 feet of unobstructed space beyond both the starting and finish lines (total of 50 feet long). Cones placed on each side of lane no more than 10 feet apart.

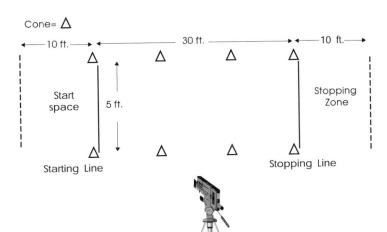

Camera Location and Operation:

Set up camera outside cones, so that student can be viewed galloping from the side. The student's entire body, including the feet, must be in view and close enough to assess the form.

National Association for Sport and Physical Education, an association of the American Alliance for Health, Physical Education, Recreation and Dance

59

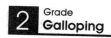

Assessment Score Sheet

PE Teacher _____ Grade _____ Date _____

School _____ Classroom Teacher _____

Student Name	ID Number	Gender	Form (0-4)	Consistency (0-4)	Total Score (0-8) 6=Competent

National Association for Sport and Physical Education, an association of the American Alliance for Health, Physical Education, Recreation and Dance

Grade

Gymnastics Sequence 2

Standard 1:

Demonstrates competency in motor skills and movement patterns needed to perform a variety of physical activities

Performance Indicator:

Create and perform a gymnastics sequence

Assessment Task:

Combine balancing, transferring weight, and rolling actions into a sequence

Criteria for Competence (Level 3):

1. Includes a momentary still beginning and ending
2. Two balances are performed and held for 3 seconds
3. Two different weight transfers are performed with good technique, one of which must be a roll

■ Assessment Rubric:

Level	1. Still Beginning and End	2. Balances	3. Weight Transfer
4	Still beginning and end are held with very clear shapes	Both balances are held for 3 seconds with good extensions	Two different weight transfers are performed smoothly with fluid motion throughout the sequence, one transfer is a roll
3	Includes a momentary still beginning and ending	2 balances are performed and held for 3 seconds	Two different weight transfers are performed with good technique, one of which must be a roll
2	Beginning or ending is not still	2 balances are performed but only 1 is held for 3 seconds	One weight transfer is performed with good technique
1	Beginning and ending are not still	Does not perform 2 balances or hold either for 3 seconds	Neither weight transfer used good technique
0	Violates safety procedures and/or does not complete the assessment task		

National Association for Sport and Physical Education, an association of the American Alliance for Health, Physical Education, Recreation and Dance

61

■ **Assessment Protocols:**

Directions for Students (Read aloud verbatim):

- Today I'm going to look at the gymnastics sequence you practiced.
- Perform your sequence the way you wrote it on your paper.
- Your sequence should include 2 different balances held for 3 seconds each and 2 different transfers of body weight, one of which is a roll (may be an egg roll or shoulder roll).
- We will be looking to see if you start your sequence in a still position and end it in a still position, and if you include all the parts of your sequence and perform your sequence smoothly.
- Start inside the rectangle and do your entire sequence inside that rectangle.

Directions for Teachers:

Preparation:

- See the manual for General Protocols for instruction, warm-up, camera location, and operation.
- Students should have designed the sequence during previous lessons and recorded the sequence on paper.
- Students should have memorized and practiced the sequence until it is repeatable.
- Clearly indicate the 10' x 20' rectangular performance area.

Safety:

- Students should only perform forward or backward rolls when they are ready. (Egg roll or shoulder roll meet the criteria.)
- Be sure students understand where to start and the boundaries of the performance area.
- Allow only safe footwear (no sandals, slides, boots, etc.).
- If outside, use a smooth surface that is free of obstructions and provide appropriate mats where needed.

Equipment/Materials:

- As many mats as necessary.

Diagram of Space/Distances:

The performance area should be limited to a 10' X 20' rectangle. You may use the floor, a floor exercise or wrestling mat, a sequence of mats, or a combination of mats and a designated space on the floor (within camera view).

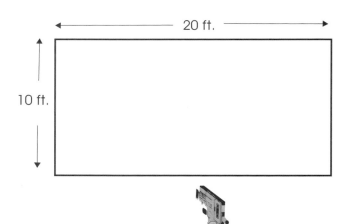

Camera Location and Operation:

The camera must be able to see the performer during the entire routine. A side view of the performer is best.

NASPE

Assessment Score Sheet

PE Teacher _____ Grade _____ Date _____

School _____ Classroom Teacher _____

Student Name	ID Number	Gender	Beginning and Ending (0-4)	Balances (0-4)	Weight Transfer (0-4)	Total Score (0-12) 9=Competent

National Association for Sport and Physical Education, an association of the American Alliance for Health, Physical Education, Recreation and Dance

63

2 Grade
Jump Forward

Standard 1:

Demonstrates competency in motor skills and movement patterns needed to perform a variety of physical activities

Performance Indicator:

Demonstrates a mature pattern of jumping, galloping, sliding, and skipping

Assessment Task:

Jump forward using a two-foot take off and a two-foot landing

Criteria for Competence (Level 3):

1. Jumps with the essential elements of a mature pattern:

   a) arms back and knees bent in preparation

   b) 2 foot simultaneous take off

   c) swing of arms forward to at least shoulder height

   d) 2 foot simultaneous landing

   e) knees bend on landing

   F) jumps with one continuous motion

2. Jumps with sufficient force to propel the body forward at least 3 feet without falling backwards

■ Assessment Rubric:

Level	1. Form	2. Distance
4	Displays all the essential elements of a mature pattern with fluid motion	Jumps with smooth, balanced action traveling forward at least 3 feet without falling backwards
3	Jumps with the essential elements of a mature pattern: a) arms back and knees bent in preparation b) 2 foot simultaneous take off c) swing of arms forward to at least shoulder height d) 2 foot simultaneous landing e) knees bend on landing f) jumps with one continuous motion	Jumps with sufficient force to propel the body forward at least 3 feet without falling backwards
2	Jumps with 5 out of 6 essential elements	Fails to jump forward at least 3 feet OR falls backwards on landing
1	Jumps with 4 or fewer essential elements	Fails to jump forward at least 3 feet AND falls backwards on landing
0	Violates safety procedures and/or does not complete the assessment task	

Note: Toes must be behind the starting line prior to the jump and feet must completely clear the jumping line when landing.

National Association for Sport and Physical Education, an association of the American Alliance for Health, Physical Education, Recreation and Dance

■ Assessment Protocols:

Directions for Students (Read aloud verbatim):

- Today I'm going to look at your jumping.
- Stand behind the starting line.
- On my signal you will jump forward at least 3 feet using a two-foot take-off and a two-foot landing without falling backwards.
- Your feet must land over the "jumping line."
- Then step back to your starting spot.
- Wait for the 'jump when ready' signal each time.
- This is not a contest to see who can jump the farthest.
- Show me your best jumping form by starting with your arms back and knees bent, jumping from two feet at the same time as you bring your arms forward as high as your shoulders, and land on two feet with a bend in your knees.
- Jump with one continuous motion.
- You will do 3 jumps.

Directions to Teachers:

Preparation

- See the manual for General Protocols for instruction, warm-up, camera location, and operation.
- Three students can be assessed at one time.
- Clearly indicate the starting and jumping lines.
- If necessary, reiterate directions to students that this is not a contest to see who can jump the farthest.

Safety:

- Be sure students understand where their starting spot is located.
- Allow only safe footwear (no sandals, slides, boots, bare feet, etc.).
- If outside, use smooth hard surface that is free of obstructions.

Equipment/Materials:

- Tape for 2 lines on floor at least 10' long
- 3 spots marked on the starting line

Diagram of Space/Distances:

Mark 3 spots on the starting line to indicate where students should start. Place the jumping line 3' away.

S=Student

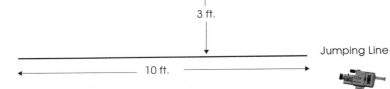

Starting Line

3 ft.

Jumping Line

10 ft.

Camera Location and Operation:

Set up camera at an angle in front of and at the end of the jumping line. It must be far enough away so that all 3 students can be viewed while jumping at the same time. The jumping line and the student's entire body, including the feet, must be in view and close enough to assess the form.

National Association for Sport and Physical Education, an association of the American Alliance for Health, Physical Education, Recreation and Dance

65

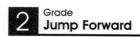

Assessment Score Sheet

PE Teacher _____ Grade _____ Date _____

School _____ Classroom Teacher _____

Student Name	ID Number	Gender	Form (0-4)			Distance (0-4)			Total Score (0-24) 18=Competent
			1st	2nd	3rd	1st	2nd	3rd	

National Association for Sport and Physical Education, an association of the American Alliance for Health, Physical Education, Recreation and Dance

Jumping & Landing Combination

Standard 1:

Demonstrates competency in motor skills and movement patterns needed to perform a variety of physical activities

Performance Indicator:

Jump and land in various combinations (one to same foot, one to the other foot, one to two feet, two to two feet, two to one foot)

Assessment Task:

From a walk or jog, jump onto a box with a 1 foot take-off, landing on 2 feet, and jump down from the box using a 2 foot take-off and landing on 2 feet

Criteria for Competence (Level 3):

1. Jumping on to a box:
   a) Makes a smooth transition into the 1 foot take off
   b) Uses a 1 foot take off
   c) Uses a 2 foot landing on the box
   d) Jumps to a controlled position on top of the box

2. Jumping off of the box:
   a) Uses a 2 foot take off
   b) Uses a 2 foot landing
   c) Absorbs the force of the landing through the feet, knees and hips
   d) Jumps to a controlled landing

■ Assessment Rubric:

Level	1. Jump On to the Box	2. Jump Off of the Box
4	Displays all the selected essential elements with fluid motion	Jumps with smooth, balanced action
3	Jumps on to box with selected criteria: a) Makes a smooth transition into the 1 foot take off b) Uses a 1 foot take off c) Uses a 2 foot landing on the box d) Jumps to a controlled position on top of the box	Jumps off box with selected criteria: a) Uses a 2 foot take off b) Uses a 2 foot landing c) Absorbs force of the landing through the feet, knees and hips d) Jumps to a controlled landing
2	Jumps with 3 essential elements present	Jumps with 3 essential elements present
1	Jumps with 2 or fewer essential elements present	Jumps with 2 or fewer essential elements present
0	Violates safety procedures and/or does not complete the assessment task	

National Association for Sport and Physical Education, an association of the American Alliance for Health, Physical Education, Recreation and Dance

67

■ **Assessment Protocols:**

Directions for Students (Read aloud verbatim):

- Today I am going to look at your jumping and landing form.

  Begin on the starting line, walk or jog to the box, and jump from one foot onto the box landing on 2 feet in a controlled position.

- You will then jump down from the box using a 2 foot take off to a 2 foot landing.

- Remember, 1 foot to 2 then 2 feet to 2. We will be looking to see if you can smoothly go into your 1 to 2 foot jump and pause and then make a good 2 foot jump with a controlled landing.

- Again, you must take off from only 1 foot and land with 2 feet on the box. Take off from the box on 2 feet and land on 2 feet.

Directions for Teachers:

Preparation:

- See the manual for General Protocols for instruction, warm-up, camera location, and operation.
- Assess one student at a time.
- Allow students to jump when they are ready.

Safety:

- Use stable boxes/low bench or mats (that do not tip or slide).
- Allow only safe footwear (no sandals, slides, boots, bare feet, etc.).
- If outside, use smooth hard surface that is free of obstructions.

Equipment/Materials:

- 1 jumping box/low benches or mat (12" high)
- 1 landing mat

Diagram of Space/Distances:

Place a starting line five feet from the box. Place mat next to the box for landing. Set up the camera so that you can see the start and mat landing for the student being tested.

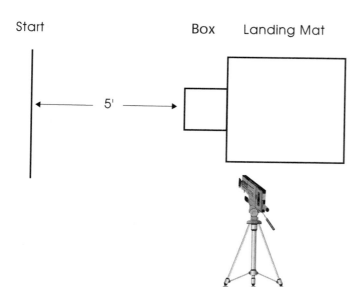

Start   Box   Landing Mat

5'

Camera Location and Operation:

Set up camera to the side of the box the student is jumping onto. The student's entire body, including the feet, must be in view and close enough to assess the form. The camera should be placed so that you can see the beginning and end of each student's performance.

Assessment Score Sheet

PE Teacher _____ Grade _____ Date _____

School _____ Classroom Teacher _____

Student Name	ID Number	Gender	Jump on to the Box (0-4)	Jump off of the Box (0-4)	Total Score (0-8) 6=Competent

National Association for Sport and Physical Education, an association of the American Alliance for Health, Physical Education, Recreation and Dance

69

2 Grade
Locomotor Sequence

Standard 1 :

Demonstrates competency in motor skills and movement patterns needed to perform a variety of physical activities

Performance Indicator:

Combine hopping, jumping, galloping, sliding, and skipping into locomotor sequences

Assessment Task:

Perform a sequence of 3 locomotor movements (hop, jump, gallop, slide, skip) with smooth transitions between each locomotor movement

Criteria for Competence (Level 3):

1. Performs 3 locomotor movements with mature patterns
2. Transitions between locomotor movements are smooth

■ Assessment Rubric:

Level	1. Locomotor Pattern	2. Transitions
4	Performs 3 locomotor movements with mature patterns and with fluid motion	Smooth fluid transitions throughout the sequence
3	Performs 3 locomotor movements with mature patterns	Transitions between locomotor movements are smooth
2	Performs 2 of 3 locomotor movements with mature patterns	One transition is not smooth
1	Performs 1 or no locomotor movements with a mature pattern	More than one transition is not smooth
0	Violates safety procedures and/or does not complete the assessment task	

National Association for Sport and Physical Education, an association of the American Alliance for Health, Physical Education, Recreation and Dance

■ Assessment Protocols:

Directions for Students (Read aloud verbatim):

- Today I'm going to look at the locomotor sequence you wrote down to perform.
- Start behind the starting line.
- Perform your sequence the way you wrote it on your paper.
- Stay in your lane.
- We are looking to see if you can perform your sequence using 3 locomotor movements with good form and two smooth transitions.
- Begin with one locomotor skill. When you reach the second set of cones change to another skill. When you reach the third set of cones change to your final skill.

Directions for Teachers:

Preparation

- See the manual for General Protocols for instruction, warm-up, camera location, and operation.
- Clearly indicate the 5' X 45' performance strip and where the change cones are located.
- Students should have memorized and practiced the sequence until it is repeatable.

Safety:

- Be sure students understand where to start and the boundaries of the performance area.
- Allow only safe footwear (no sandals, slides, boots, bare feet, etc.).
- If outside, use smooth hard surface that is free of obstructions.

Equipment/Materials:

- Tape or 6 cones to form a 5' X 45' performance strip

Diagram of Space/Distances:

Create a 5' x 45' area in which student performs sequence.
Cone= △

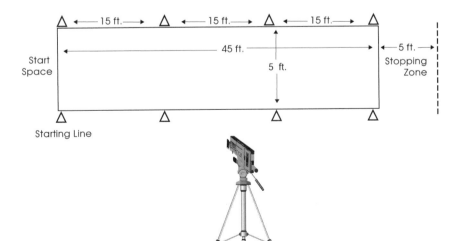

Camera Location and Operation:

Set up camera near middle of rectangular strip outside the cones, so that entire performance area can be viewed. The student's entire body, including the feet, must be in view and close enough to assess the form. Move the camera focus to be able to keep the student in the center of the picture during the whole sequence.

National Association for Sport and Physical Education, an association of the American Alliance for Health, Physical Education, Recreation and Dance

71

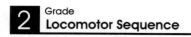 **Grade**
Locomotor Sequence

 NASPE

Assessment Score Sheet

PE Teacher _____ Grade _____ Date _____

School _____ Classroom Teacher _____

Student Name	ID Number	Gender	Locomotor Patterns (0-4)	Transitions (0-4)	Total Score (0-8) 6=Competent

National Association for Sport and Physical Education, an association of the American Alliance for Health, Physical Education, Recreation and Dance

Overhand Catching

Standard 1:

Demonstrates competency in motor skills and movement patterns needed to perform a variety of physical activities

Performance Indicator:

Dribble, kick, throw, catch, and strike a ball

Assessment Task:

Catch a ball tossed by the teacher using an overhand catching pattern

Criteria for Competency (Level 3):

1. Attempts the catch with selected essential elements:

    a) hands reach to meet the ball

    b) only hands contact the ball

    c) correct overhand catching pattern (thumbs "in")

    d) gives with the ball

2. Successfully catches the ball

■ Assessment Rubric:

Level	1. Form	2. Catches the ball
4	Display all the selected essential elements with fluid motion	Catches the ball with smooth action
3	Attempts the catch with selected essential elements: a) hands reach to meet the ball b) only hands contact the ball c) correct overhand catching pattern (thumbs "in") d) gives with the ball	Successfully catches the ball
2	Attempts the catch with 3 of 4 essential elements present	Catches the ball but then juggles the ball and recovers it
1	Attempts the catch with 2 or fewer essential elements present	Fails to catch the ball or catches then drops the ball
0	Violates safety procedures and/or does not complete the assessment task	

Note: "Attempts the catch" is used so student is given credit for mechanics regardless of success of catch. Success is measured in the "Catches the ball" category.

National Association for Sport and Physical Education, an association of the American Alliance for Health, Physical Education, Recreation and Dance

73

■ **Assessment Protocols:**

Directions for Students (Read aloud verbatim):

- Today I'm going to look at your overhand catch.
- Start on your spot, but you don't have to stay there to catch the ball.
- I will toss a ball to you.
- Show me your best overhand catching form by having your hands in ready position, reach for the ball using only your hands with your thumbs facing in, and give with the ball.
- You will have 3 tries.

Directions for Teachers:

Preparation

- See the manual for General Protocols for instruction, warm-up, camera location, and operation.
- Clearly indicate where student should stand (15' from teacher).
- Use a gentle underhand toss that gets to the student between chest and head height.
- If the toss is poor, you may repeat the toss after verbally indicating on the video that the toss will be repeated.

Safety:

- Set up catching area so that no other students can enter it.

Equipment/Materials:

- 4 playground balls (size 8-10")
- 2 spots marked on floor

Diagram of Space/Distances:

Mark two spots on the floor 15' apart. Teacher stands on one and student on the other spot. Student faces away from any distractions.

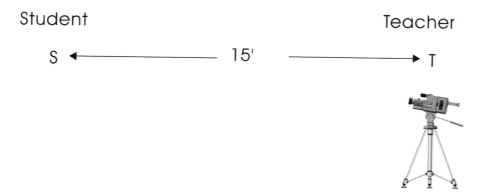

Student   Teacher

S ← ———— 15' ———— → T

Camera Location and Operation:

Set up camera beside the teacher so that it points directly toward the student. The student's entire body, including the feet, must be in view and close enough to assess the form.

74

National Association for Sport and Physical Education, an association of the American Alliance for Health, Physical Education, Recreation and Dance

Assessment Score Sheet

PE Teacher _____   Grade _____   Date _____

School _____   Classroom Teacher _____

Student Name Ball	ID Number	Gender	Form (0-4)			Catches the (0-4)			Total Score (0-24) 18=Competent
			1st	2nd	3rd	1st	2nd	3rd	

National Association for Sport and Physical Education, an association of the American Alliance for Health, Physical Education, Recreation and Dance

75

2 Grade
Skipping

Standard 1:

Demonstrates competency in motor skills and movement patterns needed to perform a variety of physical activities

Performance Indicator:

Demonstrates a mature pattern of jumping, galloping, sliding, and skipping

Assessment Task:

Skip continuously for 30 feet

Criteria for Competence (Level 3):

1. Skips with the essential elements of a mature pattern:

    a) step-hop action on alternating feet

    b) moment of non-support

2. Skips a distance of 30 feet with no breaks in movement or loss of balance

■ Assessment Rubric:

Level	1. Form	2. Consistency
4	Displays all the essential elements of a mature pattern with fluid motion	Skips with smooth movement for 30 feet

3	Skips with the essential elements of a mature pattern:
	    a) step-hop action on alternating feet
	    b) moment of non-support
		Skips for 30 feet with no breaks in movement or loss of balance

2	Skips with 1 of 2 essential elements present	Skips for 30 feet with no more than 1 break in movement or loss of balance
1	Lacks the essential elements of skipping	Skips for less than 30 feet, or with 2 or more breaks in movement, or loses balance
0	Violates safety procedures and/or does not complete the assessment task	

National Association for Sport and Physical Education, an association of the American Alliance for Health, Physical Education, Recreation and Dance

■ **Assessment Protocols:**

Directions for Students (Read aloud verbatim):

- Today I'm going to look at your skipping.
- Stand behind the starting line.
- Skip from the starting line to the finish line while staying in your lane.
- This is not a race.
- Show me your best skipping form by using a step-hop action with alternating feet and no breaks in the movement.
- On my signal, skip to the finish line.

Directions for Teachers:

Preparation

- See the manual for General Protocols for instruction, warm-up, camera location, and operation.
- Clearly indicate the lane area and finish line.

Safety:

- Be sure students understand where the finish line is located.
- Allow only safe footwear (no sandals, boots, bare feet, etc.).
- If outside, use smooth hard surface that is free of obstructions.

Equipment/Materials:

- At least 8 cones to form lane
- Mark the floor to form starting line and finish line

Diagram of Space/Distances:

Use cones to form a lane 5 feet wide and 30 feet long with an additional 10 feet of unobstructed space beyond both the starting and finish lines (total of 50 feet long). Cones placed on each side of lane 10 feet apart.

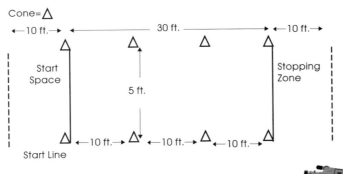

Camera Location and Operation:

Set up camera near end of lane but outside cones, so that student can be viewed the entire 30 feet. The student's entire body, including feet, must be in view and close enough to assess form.

National Association for Sport and Physical Education, an association of the American Alliance for Health, Physical Education, Recreation and Dance

77

Assessment Score Sheet

PE Teacher _____ Grade _____ Date _____

School _____ Classroom Teacher _____

Student Name	ID Number	Gender	Form (0-4)	Consistency (0-4)	Total Score (0-8) 6=Competent

National Association for Sport and Physical Education, an association of the American Alliance for Health, Physical Education, Recreation and Dance

Standard 1:

Demonstrates competency in motor skills and movement patterns needed to perform a variety of physical activities

Performance Indicator:

Dribble, kick, throw, catch, and strike a ball

Assessment Task:

Strike a ball upward 5 times consecutively with a short-handled paddle

Criteria for Competence (Level 3):

1. Strikes the ball for 5 continuous hits
2. Does not move outside the 10 foot square

■ Assessment Rubric:

Level	1. Success	2. Control
4	Strikes the ball for more than 5 continuous hits	Very little travel from the starting position
3	Strikes the ball for 5 continuous hits	Does not move outside the 10 foot square
2	Strikes for 3 or 4 continuous hits	Moves outside the boundaries 1 or 2 times within the time frame
1	Strikes for 1 hit or 2 continuous hits	Moves outside the boundaries 3 or more times within the time frame
0	Violates safety procedures and/or does not complete the assessment task	

National Association for Sport and Physical Education, an association of the American Alliance for Health, Physical Education, Recreation and Dance

79

■ **Assessment Protocols:**

Directions for Students (Read aloud verbatim):

- Today I'm going to watch you striking a ball upward.
- You will have 30 seconds to try as many times as you can to get 5 or more hits in a row.
- Stand in the center of your personal space area and stay in your area.
- Try to strike the ball at least 5 times in a row staying in your area.
- If the ball hits the floor, bring it to the center of your space and start again.

Directions for Teachers:

Preparation

- See the manual for General Protocols for instruction, warm-up, camera location, and operation.
- Clearly indicate the personal space area.
- The trial ends when the student has struck the ball 5 or more times consecutively OR 30 seconds has elapsed, whichever occurs first.
- Have another ball available for student in case first ball gets away.

Safety:

- Be sure students understand where their personal space area is located.
- If outside, use smooth hard surface that is free of obstructions.

Equipment/Materials:

- Short wooden or plastic paddle (not a racket with strings)
- Baseball sized or tennis ball sized soft foam ball
- Floor tape or cones
- Stopwatch or clock for timing 30 seconds

Diagram of Space/Distances:

Mark a 10 ft. by 10 ft. square by using tape or cones.

Cone= △

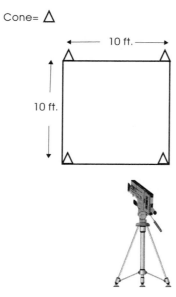

10 ft.

10 ft.

Camera Location and Operation:

Set up camera in front of the student and far enough away so that the entire personal space area can be viewed. The student's entire body, including the feet, must be in view and close enough to assess the form.

Assessment Score Sheet

PE Teacher _____ Grade _____ Date _____

School _____ Classroom Teacher _____

Student Name	ID Number	Gender	Success (0-4)	Control (0-4)	Total Score (0-8) 6=Competent

National Association for Sport and Physical Education, an association of the American Alliance for Health, Physical Education, Recreation and Dance

81

National Association for Sport and Physical Education, an association of the American Alliance for Health, Physical Education, Recreation and Dance

Grade

Basketball: Defense 5

Standard 1:

Demonstrates competency in motor skills and movement patterns needed to perform a variety of physical activities

Performance Indicator:

Use defensive skills to gain possession of an object in a 2 on 1 situation

Assessment Task:

Gain possession of a basketball in a 2 on 1 situation

Criteria for Competence: (Level 3)

1. Usually assumes defensive stance while guarding:
   a) wide base of support
   b) hands in a ready position
2. Usually moves to block off the passing lane
3. Usually plays aggressive defense by intercepting or making passing difficult for the offensive players

■ Assessment Rubric:

Level	1. Defensive Stance	2. Blocks Passing Lanes	3. Aggressive Defense
4	Consistently assumes defensive stance while guarding	Consistently moves to block off the passing lane	Consistently plays aggressive defense by intercepting or making passing difficult for the offensive players
3	Usually assumes defensive stance while guarding a) wide base of support b) hands in a ready position	Usually moves to block off the passing lane	Usually plays aggressive defense by intercepting or making passing difficult for the offensive players
2	Sometimes assumes defensive stance while guarding	Sometimes moves to block off the passing lane	Sometimes plays aggressive defense by intercepting or making passing difficult for the offensive players
1	Seldom assumes defensive stance while guarding	Seldom moves to block off the passing lane	Seldom plays aggressive defense by intercepting or making passing difficult for the offensive players
0	Violates safety procedures and/or does not complete the assessment task		

Consistently = above 90%

Usually = 75% - 89%

Sometimes = 50% -74%

Seldom = below 50%

National Association for Sport and Physical Education, an association of the American Alliance for Health, Physical Education, Recreation and Dance

83

■ **Assessment Protocols:**

Directions for Students (Read aloud verbatim):

- You will try to gain possession of a basketball against 2 offensive players who will attempt to keep the ball away from you.
- You will play for 1 minute.
- You will be assessed on your ability to:
  a) Assume a good defensive stance while guarding by using a wide base of support and having your hands in a ready position;
  b) Move to block off the passing lane;
  c) Play aggressive defense by intercepting or making passing difficult for the offensive players.
- The offensive players will start the ball. If the defense gets the ball, give the ball back to the offense.

Directions for Teachers:

Preparation

- See the manual for General Protocols for instruction, warm-up, camera location, and operation.
- Select several competent students to alternate as offensive players. Instruct offensive players to play aggressively.

Safety:

- Playing area must be dry and clean with at least 3 feet of clear space beyond the boundary line.

Equipment:

- Marked playing area (30' X 30')
- Youth Basketball
- Stopwatch

Diagram of space/distance:

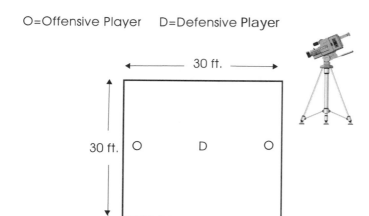

O=Offensive Player   D=Defensive Player

Camera Location/Operation:

The camera should be placed at a corner with sufficient distance to see all boundary lines within the viewing screen.

NASPE

Assessment Score Sheet

PE Teacher _____ Grade _____ Date _____

School _____ Classroom Teacher _____

Student Name	ID Number	Gender	Defensive Stance (0-4)	Block Passing Lane (0-4)	Aggressive Defense (0-4)	Total Score (0-12) 9=Competent

5 Soccer: Dribble, Pass and Receive

Grade

Standard 1:

Demonstrates competence in motor skills and movement patterns needed to perform a variety of physical activities

Performance Indicator:

Dribble, pass, and receive a ball with a partner

Assessment Task:

Dribble, pass, and receive a soccer ball while traveling at a jog

Criteria for Competence (Level 3):

1. Dribble with control while moving at a slow consistent jog
2. Sends a receivable lead pass to a partner so it can be received outside the passing lane without a break in the receiver's stride on at least 3 passes
3. Moves forward and outside the passing lane to meet the ball while receiving at least 3 receivable passes

■ Assessment Rubric:

Level	1. Dribbling	2. Passing	3. Receiving
4	Dribbles with consistent rhythm and control while moving at a slow consistent jog	Sends a receivable lead pass to a partner so it can be received outside the passing lane without a break in the receiver's stride on all 4 passes	Moves forward and outside the passing lane to receive 4 receivable passes
3	Dribbles with control while moving at a slow consistent jog	Sends a receivable lead pass to a partner so it can be received outside the passing lane without a break in the receiver's stride on at least 3 passes	Moves forward and outside the passing lane to meet the ball while receiving at least 3 receivable passes
2	Dribbles with control while moving at an inconsistent or slow speed	Sends a receivable lead pass outside the passing lane to a partner so it can be received without a break in the receiver's stride on 2 passes	Moves forward to receive at least 2 receivable passes
1	Dribbles with frequent lack of control and/or inconsistent walking or jogging speed	Sends a receivable lead pass outside the passing lane to a partner so it can be received without a break in the receiver's stride on fewer than 2 passes	Moves to receive fewer than 2 receivable passes
0	Violates safety procedures and/or does not complete the assessment task		

Assessment Protocols:

Directions for Students (Read aloud verbatim and provide a visual demonstration without the ball):

- You and your partner will perform dribbling, passing, and receiving skills while traveling on the outside of a passing lane marked by polyspots.
- The first person with the ball will dribble a short distance and then pass to a partner. You need to get the ball to your partner ahead of them and outside the passing lane. The person receiving the ball will dribble and then pass the ball back to the first person. Continue this pattern so that each person completes 2 passes and 2 receptions. If you need to move inside the passing lane to receive the ball, dribble it back to the outside of the passing lane before you pass it to your partner. When you reach the end line, turn around and repeat the passes coming back. Each of you will complete a total of at least 4 passes (2 going up, 2 coming back).
- You will be assessed on your ability to:
  a) Dribble with control while moving at a slow jog;
  b) Send a receivable lead pass to your partner;
  c) Move to receive a receivable pass.

Directions for Teachers:

Preparation

- See the manual for General Protocols for instruction, warm-up, camera location, and operation.
- Students of relatively equal skill determined by prior assessment should be paired together.

Safety:

- Area should be mowed and be free of obstructions.

Equipment:

- 8 polyspots or 4" cones
- Lane marked 15 ft by 150 ft
- Appropriate size soccer ball

Diagram of space/distance – mark camera location

A=Player A-Starting position   B=Player B-Starting Position
▲=Polyspots mark passing lane (Passing lane=15 ft wide and approximately 150 ft long).
Path of Player B= ▬▬▬▬▬▬
Path of Ball= - - - - - - ►
Path of Player A= ▬ ▬ ▬ ▬
Starting Line= ▬▬▬▬

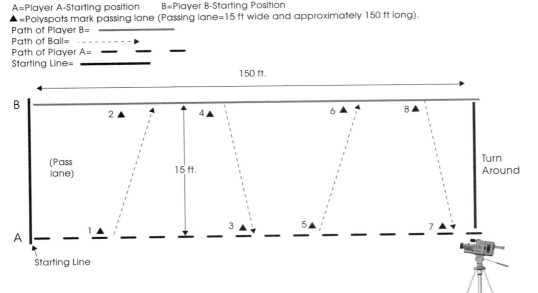

Camera Location/Operation

The camera should be placed to the side of the end line so that the players can be viewed for the entire distance to be traveled. The beginning line should be seen at the top and the end line at the bottom of the viewing screen.

National Association for Sport and Physical Education, an association of the American Alliance for Health, Physical Education, Recreation and Dance

87

Assessment Score Sheet

PE Teacher _____   Grade _____   Date _____

School _____   Classroom Teacher _____

Student Name	ID Number	Gender	Dribbling (0-4)	Passing (0-4)	Receiving (0-4)	Total Score (0-12) 9=Competent

Grade

Soccer: Offense **5**

Standard 1:

Demonstrates competence in motor skills and movement patterns needed to perform a variety of physical activities

Performance Indicator:

Use offensive skills to maintain possession of an object in a 2 on 1 situation

Assessment Task:

Use offensive skills to maintain possession of the ball in a 2 on 1 game of soccer

Criteria for Competence (Level 3):

1. Usually moves to create open space and a passing lane
2. Usually sends a receivable lead pass to a teammate
3. Usually receives a receivable pass and controls ball

■ Assessment Rubric:

Level	1. Movement Without the Ball	2. Passing	3. Receiving
4	Consistently moves to create open space and a passing lane	Consistently sends a receivable lead pass to a teammate	Consistently receives a receivable pass and controls ball
3	Usually moves to create open space and a passing lane	Usually sends a receivable lead pass to a teammate	Usually receives a receivable pass and controls ball
2	Sometimes moves to create open space and a passing lane	Sometimes sends a receivable lead pass to a teammate	Sometimes receives a receivable pass and controls ball
1	Seldom moves to create open space and a passing lane	Seldom sends a receivable lead pass to a teammate	Seldom receives a receivable pass and controls ball
0	Violates safety procedures and/or does not complete the assessment task		

Consistently = above 90%

Usually = 75% - 89%

Sometimes = 50% - 74%

Seldom = below 50%

National Association for Sport and Physical Education, an association of the American Alliance for Health, Physical Education, Recreation and Dance

89

■ **Assessment Protocols:**

Directions for Students (Read aloud verbatim):

- You and your partner will play a 2 on 1 game of soccer against a defender for 1 minute.
- You will be assessed on your ability to:
  a) Move to create open space and passing lanes;
  b) Send receivable passes;
  c) Receive receivable passes.
- All passes must be leading passes, so that the receiver must move to the ball.
- One partner will start play. Each time play is interrupted, play will be resumed alternating the initiator.

Directions for Teachers:

Preparation

- See the manual for General Protocols for instruction, warm-up, camera location, and operation.
- Students of relatively equal skill determined by prior assessment should be paired together.
- Select several students to alternate as the defensive player. Instruct defender to moderately restrict, obstruct or intercept passes.
- One partner will start play. Each time play is interrupted play will be resumed alternating the initiator.

Safety:

- Fields should be mowed short, level and free from holes and obstruction.

Equipment:

- Marked field
- Soccer ball
- 4 cones
- Pinnies/jerseys of a contrasting color
- Stopwatch

Diagram of space/distance

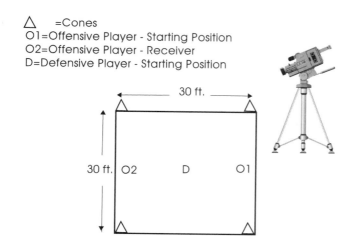

△ = Cones
O1 = Offensive Player - Starting Position
O2 = Offensive Player - Receiver
D = Defensive Player - Starting Position

30 ft.

30 ft.

O2   D   O1

Camera Location/Operation:

The camera should be placed at a corner with sufficient distance to see all boundary lines within the viewing screen.

90

National Association for Sport and Physical Education, an association of the American Alliance for Health, Physical Education, Recreation and Dance

Assessment Score Sheet

PE Teacher _____ Grade _____ Date _____

School _____ Classroom Teacher _____

Student Name	ID Number	Gender	Movement without the Ball (0-4)	Passing (0-4)	Receiving (0-4)	Total Score (0-12) 9=Competent

National Association for Sport and Physical Education, an association of the American Alliance for Health, Physical Education, Recreation and Dance

91

5 Grade Dance

Standard 1:

Demonstrates competency in motor skills and movement patterns needed to perform a variety of physical activities

Performance Indicator:

Perform a dance

Assessment Task:

Perform the given steps and sequences to the beat of the music for an age appropriate dance (e.g. line, square, folk, step, social)

Criteria for Competence (Level 3):

1. Consistently performs steps of the dance correctly
2. Consistently performs sequences of the dance correctly
3. Consistently moves to the beat of the music

■ Assessment Rubric:

Level	1. Steps	2. Sequences	3. Beat of the Music
4	Always performs steps (movements, space, position) of the dance correctly	Always performs sequences (movement sequences, order) of the dance correctly	Always moves to the beat of the music
3	Consistently performs steps of the dance correctly	Consistently performs sequences of the dance correctly	Consistently moves to the beat of the music
2	Usually performs steps of the dance correctly	Usually performs sequences of the dance correctly	Usually moves to the beat of the music
1	Sometimes or never performs steps of the dance correctly	Sometimes or never performs sequences of the dance correctly	Sometimes or never moves to the beat of the music
0	Violates safety procedures and/or does not complete the assessment task		

Always = no errors

Consistently = 90% or above

Usually = 75% - 89%

Sometimes or never = below 75%

■ **Assessment Protocols:**

Directions for Students (Read aloud verbatim):

- You will perform a dance we have learned and practiced.
- You will be assessed on your ability to:
    - a) perform the steps of the dance;
    - b) perform the sequences of the dance;
    - c) consistently move to the beat of the music.
- Continue dance until the music stops.

Directions for Teachers:

Preparation

- See the manual for General Protocols for instruction, warm-up, camera location, and operation.
- The teacher selects an age-appropriate dance from those that students have been taught and have practiced.
- The dance selected should be representative of the steps most common among the dances taught.
- Instrumental music is recommended unless verbal direction (as in square dance) is included on recording.
- Students should be spaced so that each can be clearly seen by the teacher and the camera.
- Group students with a partner or in a small group as may be required for your dance.
- Continue music until the end of the "song" or play for 2 minutes.

Safety:

- Dance area is clean and dry, free from obstruction with clear perimeter around the dance area.

Equipment:

- CD/Tape player
- CD or tape
- See Appendix for grade-level appropriate dances and resources

Diagram of space/distance:

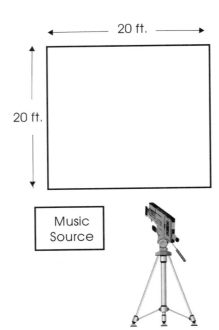

Camera Location/Operation:

The camera can be placed in front of the dancers so that all can be seen in the viewing screen. The music source must be close enough to the camera to that the music can also be recorded.

National Association for Sport and Physical Education, an association of the American Alliance for Health, Physical Education, Recreation and Dance

93

Assessment Score Sheet

PE Teacher _____   Grade _____   Date _____

School _____   Classroom Teacher _____

Student Name	ID Number	Gender	1. Steps (0-4)	2. Sequences (0-4)	3. Beat of the Music (0-4)	Total Score (0-12) 9=Competent

Grade
Floor Hockey: Dribble & Shoot 5

Standard 1:
Demonstrates competency in motor skills and movement patterns needed to perform a variety of physical activities

Performance Indicator:
Dribble and shoot an object for a goal

Assessment Task:
While jogging, continuously dribble a puck with a hockey stick through a zigzag obstacle course, and shoot for a goal

Criteria for Competence (Level 3):
1. Dribbles the hockey puck with essential elements:
   a) grip of hockey stick with dominant hand lower, thumbs pointing to ground, hands apart
   b) continuous dribble
   c) uses both sides of stick
   d) maintains slow jog
2. Shoots using all essential elements:
   a) sets up for shot by trapping or controlling the puck
   b) uses a push shot
   c) follows through to target

■ Assessment Rubric:

Level	1. Dribble	2. Shoot
4	Displays all the essential elements with fluid motion	Shoots using all the essential elements with fluid motion
3	Dribbles the hockey puck with all essential elements: a) grip of hockey stick with dominant hand lower, thumbs pointing to ground, hands apart b) continuous dribble* c) uses both sides of stick d) maintains slow jog	Shoots using all the essential elements a) sets up for shot by trapping or controlling the puck b) uses a push shot c) follows through to target
2	Dribbles with 3 of 4 essential elements present	Shoots using 2 of 3 essential elements
1	Dribbles with 2 or fewer essential elements present	Shoots using only 1 of 3 of the essential elements
0	Violates safety procedures and/or does not complete the assessment task	

*Puck should be kept within 4 feet of stick

National Association for Sport and Physical Education, an association of the American Alliance for Health, Physical Education, Recreation and Dance

95

■ **Assessment Protocols:**

Directions for Students (Read aloud verbatim):

- Today I'm going to watch you dribble and shoot for a goal using a hockey stick.
- Stand behind the starting line.
- On my signal, dribble the puck in and out of the 3 cones within the side boundaries while you jog slowly.
- Trap the puck when necessary to keep it from going outside the boundaries.
- This is not a race.
- When you reach the shooting line, first trap or control the puck, then shoot for the goal.
- Show me your best dribbling, trapping, and shooting form.

Directions for Teachers:

Preparation

- See the manual for General Protocols for instruction, warm-up, camera location, and operation.
- Clearly indicate the start, dribbling course, shooting line, and goal.
- Assessment is 1 trial.
- Intent of assessment is the dribble, trapping or controlling the puck, and shooting, not scoring a goal.

Safety:

- Set up course so that no other students can enter.
- Place goal near a wall so that shots do not interfere with other students.
- Allow only safe footwear (no sandals, boots, bare feet, etc.).
- If outside, use smooth hard surface that is free of obstructions.

Equipment/Materials:

- 1 hockey stick
- 1 hockey puck
- 6 cones
- Tape for starting and shooting lines
- Poly spots or tape for marking the side lines

Diagram of Space/Distances:

Place 3 cones 15' apart to form a course 10' wide and 50' long. The first cone is 10' from the start line and the last cone is 10' from the shooting line. Use 2 cones to make a 10' wide goal 10' from the shooting line. Use poly spots or tape to mark the sidelines.

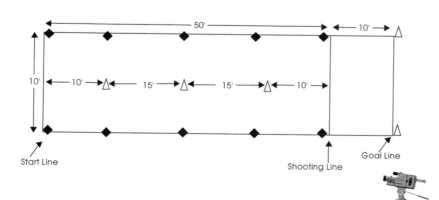

△ =Cones marking goal line and course

◆ =Polyspots marking sidelines

Camera Location and Operation:

Set up camera next to goal, so that student can be viewed dribbling, trapping, and making the shot. The student's entire body, including the feet, must be in view and close enough to assess the form.

Assessment Score Sheet

PE Teacher _____ Grade _____ Date _____

School _____ Classroom Teacher _____

Student Name	ID Number	Gender	Dribble (0-4)	Shoot (0-4)	Total Score (0-8) 6=Competent

5 Grade
Gymnastics

Standard 1:
Demonstrates competency in motor skills and movement patterns needed to perform a variety of physical activities

Performance Indicator:
Perform a gymnastics/movement sequence

Assessment Task:
Perform a self-designed gymnastics/movement sequence with the following 7 components: (1) a starting shape, (2) roll, (3) transfer of weight from feet to hands, (4) balance, (5) leap or jump, (6) turn, and (7) ending shape

Criteria for Competence (Level 3):
1. Sequence includes at least 6 of the required components
2. At least 5 of 7 components of the sequence are performed with good technique: clear beginning and ending shapes, still balances, controlled rolls, smooth weight transfers and strong leaps, jumps and turns
3. Sequence includes smooth transitions between components with no more than 2 breaks in continuity

■ Assessment Rubric:

Level	1. Composition	2. Technique	3. Transitions
4	Sequence includes all the required components	Performs 6 of 7 components with good technique	Sequence includes smooth transitions between components with no more than 1 break in continuity
3	Sequence includes 6 of the required components	Performs at least 5 of 7 components of the sequence with good technique: clear beginning and ending shapes, still balances, controlled rolls, smooth weight transfers, and strong leaps, jumps and turns	Sequence includes smooth transitions between components with no more than 2 breaks in continuity
2	Sequence includes 5 of the required components	Only 4 of the components are performed with good technique	Sequence includes transitions between components with no more than 3 breaks in continuity
1	Sequence includes 4 or fewer of the required components	Sequence includes 3 or fewer components performed with good technique	Sequence includes 4 or more breaks in continuity
0	Violates safety procedures and/or does not complete the assessment task		

■ Assessment Protocols:

Directions for Students (Read aloud verbatim):

- Perform your gymnastics/movement sequence (routine) that includes the following required components: (1) a starting shape, (2) roll, (3) transfer of weight from feet to hands, (4) balance, (5) leap or jump, (6) turn, and (7) ending shape.
- You will be assessed on your ability to:
  a) perform the sequence with good technique, clear beginning and ending shapes, still balances, controlled rolls, smooth weight transfers, and strong leaps, jumps and turns;
  b) perform all the required components;
  c) perform the sequence so that movements flow together with smooth transitions.

Directions for Teachers:

Preparation

- See the manual for General Protocols for instruction, warm-up, camera location, and operation.
- It is recommended that written routines be submitted, reviewed and approved by the teacher prior to the assessment performance.

Safety:

- Performance area must be matted, sections taped, clean and dry, free from obstruction including at least a 5 ft clear perimeter.
- Students **must** wear clothing that neither restricts nor hinders movement.
- All jewelry that could potentially injure the students as well as objects in pockets are to be removed.

Equipment:

- 20 X 20 tumbling mat (if sections of mat are used they must be taped together)
- A different placement of mats may be used to accommodate the routine, facility, or available mats (i.e., a long line of mats)

Diagram of space/distance

S=Student
M=Music Source

Camera Location/Operation:

The camera needs to be placed so that the entire performance of both performers can be seen. Camera placement will vary with mat placement and camera capability. For a 20 X 20 mat the best place for the camera will be in front (as shown) so that all corners of the area can be seen in the camera lens. For mats placed in a row the best placement will be to the side of the mats so the first and last mat can be seen within the camera angle and performers can be viewed slightly from the side.

National Association for Sport and Physical Education, an association of the American Alliance for Health, Physical Education, Recreation and Dance

99

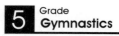

Assessment Score Sheet

PE Teacher _____   Grade _____   Date _____

School _____   Classroom Teacher _____

Student Name	ID Number	Gender	Composition (0-4)	Technique (0-4)	Transition (0-4)	Total Score (0-12) 9=Competent

National Association for Sport and Physical Education, an association of the American Alliance for Health, Physical Education, Recreation and Dance

Standard 1:

Demonstrates competency in motor skills and movement patterns needed to perform a variety of physical activities

Performance Indicator:

Perform sport specific skills for participation in individual non-competitive activities

Assessment Task:

Inline skate on a level surface with changes in direction

Criteria for Competence (Level 3):

1) Displays essential elements of forward stride without falling:
   a) short continuous strokes
   b) push sideward
   c) glide through ready position
   d) swing arms in opposition to foot stroke

2) Displays essential elements of changing direction:
   a) glide through turn at consistent speed
   b) look in direction of turn
   c) lead with inside skate

3) Displays essential elements of stopping:
   a) shoulders forward
   b) weight on non-braking leg
   c) slide brake foot forward with heel down and come to a complete stop

■ Assessment Rubric:

Level	1. Forward Stride	2. Changing Direction	3. Stopping
4	Displays all essential elements of forward stride with fluid motion without falling	Displays all essential elements of changing direction with fluid motion	Displays all essential elements of stopping to come to a complete stop with good control
3	Displays essential elements of forward stride without falling: a) short continuous strokes b) push sideward c) glide through ready position d) swing arms in opposition to foot stroke	Displays essential elements of changing direction: a) glide through turn at consistent speed b) look in direction of turn c) lead with inside skate	Displays essential elements of stopping: a) shoulders forward b) weight on non-braking leg c) slide brake foot forward with heel down and come to a complete stop
2	Displays 3 of 4 essential elements of forward stride without falling	Displays 2 of 3 essential elements of changing direction	Displays 2 of 3 essential elements of stopping
1	Displays 2 or fewer essential elements of forward stride and/or falls	Displays 1 or no essential elements of changing direction	Displays 1 or no essential elements of stopping and/or falls when stopping
0	Violates safety procedures and/or does not complete the assessment task		

National Association for Sport and Physical Education, an association of the American Alliance for Health, Physical Education, Recreation and Dance

101

■ **Assessment Protocols:**

Directions for Students (Read aloud verbatim):

- You will skate the course as marked by the cones.
- You will be assessed on your ability to:

  a) skate forward using short strokes, pushing sideward, gliding through ready position, swinging arms in opposition to foot stroke;

  b) negotiate turn at consistent speed;

  c) come to a complete stop within the stop zone with shoulders forward, weight on non-braking leg, sliding brake foot forward with heel down.

- Use short continuous strokes – no walking.
- You will go around the course twice.

Directions to Teachers: Preparation

- See the manual for General Protocols for instruction, warm-up, camera location, and operation.
- Set up the course on a basketball court or smooth surface parking lot, using cones to mark the starting, turning and stopping points.
- Students should use short continuous strokes – no walking.

Safety:

- Properly fitting skates and safety equipment (helmet, knee, wrist and elbow pads) must be worn by each student.
- Skate course must be clear of debris, holes and obstacles.
- All skates and safety equipment must be well maintained and in good working order.

Equipment:

- Properly fitting skates and safety equipment (helmet, knee, wrist and elbow pads) for each student
- 8 cones to mark start line, stop zone, skating area, and turning points
- Arrows to be taped onto cones to mark direction the student is to skate through the course

Diagram of space/distance

Course = 60 ft x 30 ft with 10 feet clear of end cones for turn
◆ = Cones

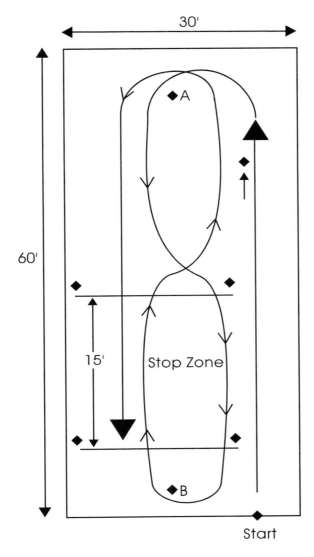

30'

60'

15'

Stop Zone

◆A

◆B

Start

Travel in a Figure 8 Pattern. Skate to Cone A and glide around to the left. On the return, cross over and glide around Cone B to the right. Return to Cone A and glide around Cone A again to the left. Skate to the Stop Zone and finish.

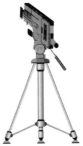

Camera Location/Operation:
Set the camera near the start/ stop zone so the stop zone can be viewed. The course and the student should be visible in the viewing screen so that performance can be clearly seen.

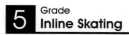

5 Grade
Inline Skating

NASPE

Assessment Score Sheet

PE Teacher _____ Grade _____ Date _____

School _____ Classroom Teacher _____

Student Name	ID Number	Gender	Forward Stride (0-4)	Changing Directions (0-4)	Stop (0-4)	Total Score (0-12) 9=Competent

Grade
Overhand Throwing 5

Standard 1:

Demonstrates competency in motor skills and movement patterns needed to perform a variety of physical activities

Performance Indicator:

Dribble, kick, throw, catch, and strike a ball

Assessment Task:

Use an overhand throwing pattern to send a ball to a large wall target

Criteria for Competence (Level 3):

1. Throws a ball with selected essential elements:

   a) throwing elbow shoulder high, hand back, and side orientation in preparation for throw

   b) trunk rotation with elbow lagging behind hip

   c) weight transfer to non-throwing forward foot

2. Hits target area on wall

■ Assessment Rubric:

Level	1. Form	2. Accuracy to Target
4	Displays all the selected essential elements with fluid motion and differentiated trunk rotation	Hits target area on wall with force
3	Throws with selected essential elements: a) throwing elbow shoulder high, hand back, and side orientation in preparation for the throw b) trunk rotation with elbow lagging behind hip c) weight transfer to non-throwing forward foot	Hits target area on wall
2	Throws with 2 of 3 essential elements	Hits wall but not target area
1	Throws with 1 or no essential elements	Ball fails to reach the wall
0	Violates safety procedures and/or does not complete the assessment task	

Note: Failure to use the overhand throwing pattern is scored as Incomplete Assessment Task

■ **Assessment Protocols:**

Directions for Students (Read aloud verbatim):

- Today I'm going to look at your overhand throw.
- You will be assessed on:
  a) having a side orientation;
  b) a good arm position;
  c) good trunk rotation;
  d) a step to your non-throwing forward foot;
  e) whether you hit the target.
- Stand behind the throwing line.
- You will have 3 trials.

Directions for Teachers:

Preparation

- See the manual for General Protocols for instruction, warm-up, camera location, and operation.
- Clearly indicate the target square on the wall and the throwing line.

Safety:

- Set up throwing area so that no other students can enter it.

Equipment/Materials:

- Tennis balls
- Tape to form throwing line and target square on a wall

Diagram of Space/Distances:

Use tape to form a throwing line on the floor and a target square 6' x 6' on a wall 25' from the throwing line. Place target square 3 feet off the floor.

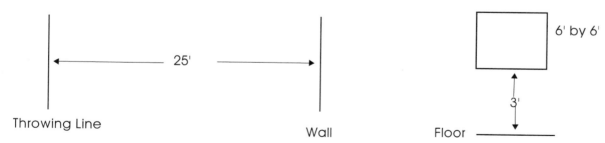

Throwing Line   Wall   Floor

25'   6' by 6'   3'

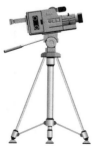

Camera Location and Operation:

Set up camera on same side as student's throwing arm. The student's entire body, including the feet, must be in view and close enough to assess the form. The camera placement should also allow the target on the wall to be seen in the picture.

NASPE

Assessment Score Sheet

PE Teacher _____ Grade _____ Date _____

School _____ Classroom Teacher _____

Student Name	ID Number	Gender	Form (0-4)			Accuracy to Target (0-4)			Total Score (0-24) 18=Competent
			1st	2nd	3rd	1st	2nd	3rd	

5 Grade
Soccer: Dribble, Pass and Receive

Standard 1:

Demonstrates competence in motor skills and movement patterns needed to perform a variety of physical activities

Performance Indicator:

Dribble, pass, and receive a ball with a partner

Assessment Task:

Dribble, pass, and receive a soccer ball while traveling at a jog

Criteria for Competence (Level 3):

1. Dribble with control while moving at a slow consistent jog
2. Sends a receivable lead pass to a partner so it can be received outside the passing lane without a break in the receiver's stride on at least 3 passes
3. Moves forward and outside the passing lane to meet the ball while receiving at least 3 receivable passes

■ Assessment Rubric:

Level	1. Dribbling	2. Passing	3. Receiving
4	Dribbles with consistent rhythm and control while moving at a slow consistent jog	Sends a receivable lead pass to a partner so it can be received outside the passing lane without a break in the receiver's stride on all 4 passes	Moves forward and outside the passing lane to receive 4 receivable passes
3	Dribbles with control while moving at a slow consistent jog	Sends a receivable lead pass to a partner so it can be received outside the passing lane without a break in the receiver's stride on at least 3 passes	Moves forward and outside the passing lane to meet the ball while receiving at least 3 receivable passes
2	Dribbles with control while moving at an inconsistent or slow speed	Sends a receivable lead pass outside the passing lane to a partner so it can be received without a break in the receiver's stride on 2 passes	Moves forward to receive at least 2 receivable passes
1	Dribbles with frequent lack of control and/or inconsistent walking or jogging speed	Sends a receivable lead pass outside the passing lane to a partner so it can be received without a break in the receiver's stride on fewer than 2 passes	Moves to receive fewer than 2 receivable passes
0	Violates safety procedures and/or does not complete the assessment task		

■ Assessment Protocols:

Directions for Students (Read aloud verbatim and provide a visual demonstration without the ball):

- You and your partner will perform dribbling, passing, and receiving skills while traveling on the outside of a passing lane marked by polyspots.
- The first person with the ball will dribble a short distance and then pass to a partner. You need to get the ball to your partner ahead of them and outside the passing lane. The person receiving the ball will dribble and then pass the ball back to the first person. Continue this pattern so that each person completes 2 passes and 2 receptions. If you need to move inside the passing lane to receive the ball, dribble it back to the outside of the passing lane before you pass it to your partner. When you reach the end line, turn around and repeat the passes coming back. Each of you will complete a total of at least 4 passes (2 going up, 2 coming back).
- You will be assessed on your ability to:
  a) Dribble with control while moving at a slow jog;
  b) Send a receivable lead pass to your partner;
  c) Move to receive a receivable pass.

Directions for Teachers:

Preparation

- See the manual for General Protocols for instruction, warm-up, camera location, and operation.
- Students of relatively equal skill determined by prior assessment should be paired together.

Safety:

- Area should be mowed and be free of obstructions.

Equipment:

- 8 polyspots or 4" cones
- Lane marked 15 ft by 150 ft
- Appropriate size soccer ball

Diagram of space/distance – mark camera location

A=Player A-Starting position   B=Player B-Starting Position
▲ =Polyspots mark passing lane (Passing lane=15 ft wide and approximately 150 ft long).
Path of Player B= ─────────
Path of Ball= - - - - - - - - ▶
Path of Player A= ━━ ━━ ━━
Starting Line= ━━━━

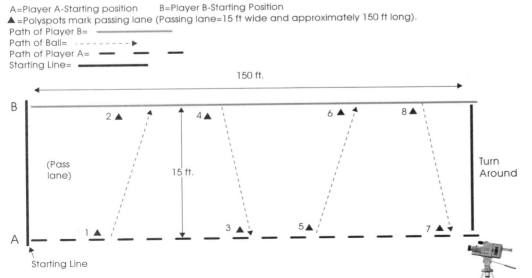

150 ft.

B

2 ▲   ▲   4 ▲   6 ▲ ▲   8 ▲

(Pass lane)   15 ft.   Turn
                                                            Around

        1 ▲   3 ▲   5 ▲   7 ▲
A ━

Starting Line

Camera Location/Operation

The camera should be placed to the side of the end line so that the players can be viewed for the entire distance to be traveled. The beginning line should be seen at the top and the end line at the bottom of the viewing screen.

National Association for Sport and Physical Education, an association of the American Alliance for Health, Physical Education, Recreation and Dance

109

Assessment Score Sheet

PE Teacher _____ Grade _____ Date _____

School _____ Classroom Teacher _____

Student Name	ID Number	Gender	Dribbling (0-4)	Passing (0-4)	Receiving (0-4)	Total Score (0-12) 9=Competent

National Association for Sport and Physical Education, an association of the American Alliance for Health, Physical Education, Recreation and Dance

Grade
Soccer: Offense 5

Standard 1:

Demonstrates competence in motor skills and movement patterns needed to perform a variety of physical activities

Performance Indicator:

Use offensive skills to maintain possession of an object in a 2 on 1 situation

Assessment Task:

Use offensive skills to maintain possession of the ball in a 2 on 1 game of soccer

Criteria for Competence (Level 3):

1. Usually moves to create open space and a passing lane
2. Usually sends a receivable lead pass to a teammate
3. Usually receives a receivable pass and controls ball

■ Assessment Rubric:

Level	1. Movement Without the Ball	2. Passing	3. Receiving
4	Consistently moves to create open space and a passing lane	Consistently sends a receivable lead pass to a teammate	Consistently receives a receivable pass and controls ball
3	Usually moves to create open space and a passing lane	Usually sends a receivable lead pass to a teammate	Usually receives a receivable pass and controls ball
2	Sometimes moves to create open space and a passing lane	Sometimes sends a receivable lead pass to a teammate	Sometimes receives a receivable pass and controls ball
1	Seldom moves to create open space and a passing lane	Seldom sends a receivable lead pass to a teammate	Seldom receives a receivable pass and controls ball
0	Violates safety procedures and/or does not complete the assessment task		

Consistently = above 90%

Usually = 75% - 89%

Sometimes = 50% - 74%

Seldom = below 50%

■ Assessment Protocols:

Directions for Students (Read aloud verbatim):

- You and your partner will play a 2 on 1 game of soccer against a defender for 1 minute.
- You will be assessed on your ability to:
  a) Move to create open space and passing lanes;
  b) Send receivable passes;
  c) Receive receivable passes.
- All passes must be leading passes, so that the receiver must move to the ball.
- One partner will start play. Each time play is interrupted, play will be resumed alternating the initiator.

Directions for Teachers:

Preparation

- See the manual for General Protocols for instruction, warm-up, camera location, and operation.
- Students of relatively equal skill determined by prior assessment should be paired together.
- Select several students to alternate as the defensive player. Instruct defender to moderately restrict, obstruct or intercept passes.
- One partner will start play. Each time play is interrupted play will be resumed alternating the initiator.

Safety:

- Fields should be mowed short, level and free from holes and obstruction.

Equipment:

- Marked field
- Soccer ball
- 4 cones
- Pinnies/jerseys of a contrasting color
- Stopwatch

Diagram of space/distance

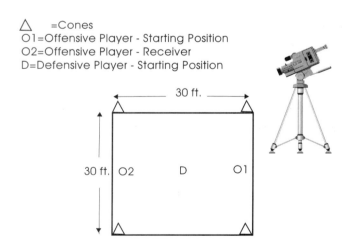

△ =Cones
O1=Offensive Player - Starting Position
O2=Offensive Player - Receiver
D=Defensive Player - Starting Position

30 ft.

30 ft. O2   D   O1

Camera Location/Operation:

The camera should be placed at a corner with sufficient distance to see all boundary lines within the viewing screen.

NASPE

Assessment Score Sheet

PE Teacher _____   Grade _____   Date _____

School _____   Classroom Teacher _____

Student Name	ID Number	Gender	Movement without the Ball (0-4)	Passing (0-4)	Receiving (0-4)	Total Score (0-12) 9=Competent

5 Grade
Striking with a Paddle

Standard 1:
Demonstrates competency in motor skills and movement patterns needed to perform a variety of physical activities

Performance Indicator:
Strike an object continuously with a paddle or racquet

Assessment Task:
Strike a ball against the wall continuously with a short-handled paddle

Criteria for Competence (Level 3):
1. Usually uses a side orientation
2. Strikes the ball continuously against the wall 5 times from 10 feet with added strokes that may be in front of the 10 foot striking line

■ Assessment Rubric:

Level	1. Form	2. Continuous Strikes
4	Consistently uses a side orientation	Strikes the ball continuously against the wall 5 times in a row from 10 feet with no hits in front of the 10 foot striking line
3	Usually uses a side orientation	Strikes the ball continuously against the wall 5 times from 10 feet with added strokes that may be in front of the 10 foot striking line
2	Sometimes uses a side orientation	Strikes the ball continuously against the wall at least 4 times from 10 feet with added strokes that may be in front of the 10 foot striking line
1	Seldom uses a side orientation	Strikes the ball continuously against the wall fewer than 4 times from 10 feet with added strokes that may be in front of the 10 foot striking line
0	Violates safety procedures and/or does not complete the assessment task	

Consistently = above 90%

Usually = 75% - 89%

Sometimes = 50% -74%

Seldom = below 50%

■ Assessment Protocols:

Directions for Students (Read aloud verbatim):

- You will strike a ball continuously, using a forehand and/or backhand stroke, against a wall, at least 5 times. Your goal is 5 good hits from behind the 10 foot line against the wall with only 1 bounce each time.
- You will be assessed on your ability to:
  a) Use a side orientation;
  b) Strike the ball continuously against the wall at least 5 times from behind the 10 foot line with added strokes that may be in front of the 10 foot striking line.
- You may strike the ball in front of the 10 foot striking line but that hit doesn't count as one of your 5 hits.
- Strike the ball after no more than 1 bounce between each contact. If the ball bounces twice, that trial is ended.
- You will have 2 opportunities to make 5 hits against the wall from behind the 10 foot line without a miss. If you do it on the first try, you don't have to do it again.
- Begin each trial by dropping the ball to bounce it prior to hitting it. Your score is counted with the hit following the first rebound from the wall.

Directions for Teachers: Preparation

- See the manual for General Protocols for instruction, warm-up, camera location, and operation.
- Trial is ended when the student fails to contact the ball before it bounces a second time, or fails to contact the ball at all. Signal the end of the trial after the 5th strike behind the 10 foot line is completed (student may not put his/her whole foot in front of the 10 foot line).
- Balls contacted in front of the 10 foot striking line are not counted.
- Students are allowed 2 trials.
- Assess 1 student at a time.

Safety:

- Courts are to be dry and free of obstruction, with adequate 10' space beyond the 10' striking line to permit forward and backward movement as needed.

Equipment:

- Floor tape for marking striking area   • 2 cones   • Pickleballs and wooden or plastic paddle

Diagram of space/distance – mark camera location

Assessment may be performed in a gymnasium or on an outdoor court against a back stop. A line 2 inches wide and 15 feet long, is to be placed 10 feet from and parallel to the wall or backstop.

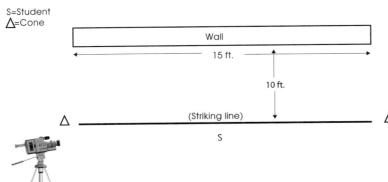

S=Student
△=Cone

Wall

← 15 ft. →

10 ft.

(Striking line)

S

(For left handers)   (For right handers)

Camera Location/Operation:
The camera can be placed to the side and slightly behind the striking line so that the length of the striking line, cones and wall and the student can be seen at the side edge of the viewing screen.

Assessment Score Sheet

PE Teacher _____   Grade _____   Date _____

School _____   Classroom Teacher _____

Student Name	ID Number	Gender	Form (0-4)	Continuous Strikes (0-4)	Total Score (0-8) 6=Competence

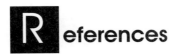

References

Hambleton, R.K., Swaminathan, H., & Rogers, J.H. (1991). Fundamentals of item response theory. Newbury Park, CA: Sage.

Kolen, M.J., & Brennan, R.L. (2004). Test equating, scaling, and linking: Methods and practices (2nd ed.). New York: Springer.

National Association for Sport and Physical Education. (1995). *Moving into the future: National standards for physical education: A guide to content and assessment.* Reston, VA: Author.

National Association for Sport and Physical Education. (2004). *Moving into the future: National standards for physical education* (2nd ed.). Reston, VA: Author.

Safrit, M.J., Zhu, W., Costa, M.G., & Zhang, L. (1992). The difficulty of sit-up tests: An empirical investigation. *Research Quarterly for Exercise and Sport, 63*(3), 277-283.

Spray, J.A. (1987). Recent developments in measurement and possible applications to the measurement of psychomotor behavior. *Research Quarterly for Exercise and Sport, 58*, 203-209.

Umar, J. (1997). Item banking. In J.P. Keeves (Ed.), *Educational research, methodology, and measurement: An international handbook* (2nd ed., pp. 923-930). New York: Elsevier Science.

Zhu, W. (1996). Should total scores from a rating scale be directly used? *Research Quarterly for Exercise and Sport, 67*(3), 363-372.

Zhu, W. (2006). Constructing tests using item response theory. In T. Wood and W. Zhu (Eds.), *Measurement Theory and Practice in Kinesiology.* pp. 53-76. Champaign, IL: Human Kinetics.

Zhu, W. (1998). Test equating: What, why, how? *Research Quarterly for Exercise and Sport, 69*, 11-23.

Zhu, W. (2001). An empirical investigation of Rasch equating of motor function tasks. *Adapted Physical Activity Quarterly, 18*(1), 72-89.

Zhu, W., & Cole, E.L. (1996). Many-faceted Rasch calibration of a gross-motor instrument. *Research Quarterly for Exercise and Sport, 67*(1), 24-34.

Zhu, W., & Safrit, M.J. (1993). The calibration of a sit-ups task using the Rasch Poisson Counts model. *The Canadian Journal of Applied Physiology, 18*(2), 207-219.

National Association for Sport and Physical Education, an association of the American Alliance for Health, Physical Education, Recreation and Dance

117

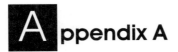# Appendix A

Dance References

Listed below are just a few samples of available materials to help teachers choose and teach dances appropriate for elementary grades.

Books

Bennett, J., & Riemer, P. (2006). *Rhythmic activities and dance* (2nd ed). Champaign, IL: Human Kinetics Publishers.

Cone, T., & Cone, S. (2006). *Teaching children dance* (2nd ed). Champaign, IL: Human Kinetics Publishers.

Mehrhof, J., & Parris, P. (2002). *And the beat goes on: Rhythmic activities for K-8.* Emporia, KS: Mirror Publishing Company.

National Association for Sport and Physical Education & National Dance Association (2007). *Teaching Dance in Elementary Physical Education.* Reston, VA: Author.

National Association for Sport and Physical Education & National Dance Association (2007). *Teaching Dance in K-12 Physical Education.* Reston, VA: Author.

Weikart, P.S. (1989). *Teaching movement and dance: A sequential approach to rhythmic movement* (3rd ed). Ypsilanti, MI: High/Scope Press.

Compact Discs available from Educational Records Center (erckids.com)

Best Dance Collection for Beginners

Best No Partner Dance Collections

Christy Lane's How to Dance Program (includes Square, Latin, African and Caribbean dances)

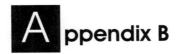

Appendix B

The NASPE National Standards for Physical Education and the Elementary Level Performance Indicators and Assessment Tasks

Standard 1:
Demonstrates competency in motor skills and movement patterns needed to perform a variety of physical activities

Kindergarten

Performance Indicator:

Throw, catch, dribble, kick, and strike from a stationary position

Assessment Task:
Continuously dribble a ball for 15 seconds with one hand

Assessment Task:
Continuously strike a balloon with a short-handled paddle using an underhand pattern for 20 seconds

Assessment Task:
Catch a ball tossed by a teacher using an underhand catching pattern

Assessment Task:
Use an underhand throwing pattern to send a ball forward through the air to a large target

Performance Indicator:

Demonstrate hopping, jumping, galloping, and sliding

Assessment Task:
Hop in place

Assessment Task:
Slide continuously for 30 feet with the preferred foot leading

Performance Indicator:

Demonstrate a mature pattern of running

Assessment Task:
Run continuously for 60 feet

Performance Indicator:

Transfer weight hands/feet

Assessment Task:

Place weight on the hands and transfer feet sideways over a raised bar and back to the starting position

Grade 2

Performance Indicator:

Dribble, kick, throw, catch, and strike a ball

Assessment Task:

Approach a stationary ball at a jog and kick with enough force to send it a distance of 30 feet on a smooth, level surface

Assessment Task:

Dribble a ball with one hand to a cone and back while jogging slowly

Assessment Task:

Catch a ball tossed by the teacher using an overhand catching pattern

Assessment Task:

Strike a ball upward 5 times consecutively with a short-handled paddle

Performance Indicator:

Perform dance sequences to music

Assessment Task:

Perform to music a grade-level appropriate individual or partner dance that utilizes 3 different patterns

Performance Indicator:

Demonstrates a mature pattern of jumping, galloping, sliding, and skipping

Assessment Task:

Gallop continuously for 30 feet with one foot leading. Repeat the task with the other foot leading

Assessment Task:

Jump forward using a two-foot take off and a two-foot landing

Assessment Task:

Perform a sequence of 3 locomotor movements (hop, jump, gallop, slide, skip) with smooth transitions between each locomotor movement

Assessment Task:

Skip continuously for 30 feet

Performance Indicator:

Create and perform a gymnastics sequence

Assessment Task:

Combine balancing, transferring weight, and rolling actions into a sequence

Performance Indicator:

Jump and land in various combinations (one to same foot, one to the other foot, one to two feet, two to two feet, two to one foot)

Assessment Task:

From a walk or jog, jump onto a box with a 1 foot take-off, landing on 2 feet, and jump down from the box using a 2 foot take-off and landing on 2 feet

Grade 5

Performance Indicator:

Use defensive skills to gain possession of an object in a 2 on 1 situation

Assessment Task:

Gain possession of a basketball in a 2 on 1 situation

Performance Indicator:

Dribble, pass, and receive a ball with a partner

Assessment Task:

Dribble, pass, and receive a basketball while traveling at a jog

Assessment Task:

Dribble, pass, and receive a soccer ball while traveling at a jog

Performance Indicator:

Use offensive skills to maintain possession of an object in a 2 on 1 situation

Assessment Task:

Maintain possession of a basketball in 2 on 1 situation against a defender

Assessment Task:

Use offensive skills to maintain possession of the ball in a 2 on 1 game of soccer

Performance Indicator:

Perform a dance

Assessment Task:

Perform the given steps and sequences to the beat of the music for an age appropriate dance (e.g. line, square, folk, step, social)

National Association for Sport and Physical Education, an association of the American Alliance for Health, Physical Education, Recreation and Dance

123

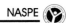

Performance Indicator:

Dribble and shoot an object for a goal

Assessment Task:

While jogging, continuously dribble a puck with a hockey stick through a zigzag obstacle course, and shoot for a goal

Performance Indicator:

Perform a gymnastics/movement sequence

Assessment Task:

Perform a self-designed gymnastics/movement sequence with the following 7 components:
(1) a starting shape, (2) roll, (3) transfer of weight from feet to hands, (4) balance, (5) leap or jump, (6) turn, and (7) ending shape

Performance Indicator:

Perform sport specific skills for participation in individual non-competitive activities

Assessment Task:

Inline skate on a level surface with changes in direction

Performance Indicator:

Dribble, kick, throw, catch, and strike a ball

Assessment Task:

Use an overhand throwing pattern to send a ball to a large wall target

Performance Indicator:

Strike an object continuously with a paddle or racquet

Assessment Task:

Strike a ball against the wall continuously with a short-handled paddle

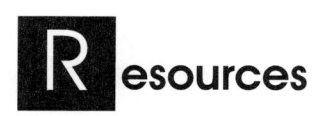

Resources

Published by the National Association for Sport and Physical Education for quality physical education programs:

Moving into the Future: National Standards for Physical Education, 2nd Edition (2004), Stock No. 304-10275

Quality Coaches, Quality Sports: National Standards for Sport Coaches, 2nd Edition (2006), Stock No. 304-10274

Movement-Based Learning: Academic Concepts and Physical Activity for Ages Three through Eight (2006), Stock No. 304-10300

Physical Educators' Guide to Successful Grant Writing (2005), Stock No. 304-10291

Physical Activity for Children: A Statement of Guidelines (2004), Stock No. 304-10276

On Your Mark… Get Set… Go!: A Guide for Beginning Physical Education Teachers (2004), Stock No. 304-10264

Concepts and Principles of Physical Education: What Every Student Needs to Know (2003), Stock No. 304-10261

Beyond Activities: Elementary Volume (2003), Stock No. 304-10265

Beyond Activities: Secondary Volume (2003), Stock No. 304-10268

National Physical Education Standards in Action (2003), Stock No. 304-10267

National Standards for Beginning Physical Education Teachers (2003), Stock No. 304-10273

Active Start: A Statement of Physical Activity Guidelines for Children Birth to Five Years (2002), Stock No. 304-10254

Appropriate Practice Documents

Appropriate Practice in Movement Programs for Young Children, (2000), Stock No. 304-10232

Appropriate Practices for Elementary School Physical Education (2000), Stock No. 304-10230

Appropriate Practices for Middle School Physical Education (2001), Stock No. 304-10248

Appropriate Practices for High School Physical Education (2004), Stock No. 304-10272

Opportunity to Learn Documents

Opportunity to Learn Standards for Elementary Physical Education (2000), Stock No. 304-10242

Opportunity to Learn Standards for Middle School Physical Education (2004), Stock No. 304-10290

Opportunity to Learn Standards for High School Physical Education (2004), Stock No. 304-10289

Assessment Series

Assessment of Swimming in Physical Education (2005), Stock No. 304-10301

Assessing Dance in Elementary Physical Education (2005), Stock No. 304-10304

Assessing Concepts: Secondary Biomechanics (2003), Stock No. 304-10220

Assessment in Outdoor Adventure Physical Education (2003), Stock No. 304-10218

Assessing Student Outcomes in Sport Education (2003), Stock No. 304-10219

Video Tools for Teaching Motor Skill Assessment (2002), Stock No. 304-10217

Assessing Heart Rate in Physical Education (2002), Stock No. 304-10214

Authentic Assessment of Physical Activity for High School Students (2002), Stock No. 304-10216

Portfolio Assessment for K-12 Physical Education (2000), Stock No. 304-10213

Elementary Heart Health: Lessons and Assessment (2001), Stock No. 304-10215

Standards-Based Assessment of Student Learning: A Comprehensive Approach (1999), Stock No. 304-10206

Assessment in Games Teaching (1999), Stock No. 304-10212

Assessing Motor Skills in Elementary Physical Education (1999), Stock No. 304-10207

Assessing and Improving Fitness in Elementary Physical Education (1999), Stock No. 304-10208

Creating Rubrics for Physical Education (1999), Stock No. 304-10209

Order online at www.naspeinfo.org or call 1-800-321-0789

Shipping and handling additional.

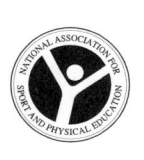

National Association for Sport and Physical Education, an association of the American Alliance for Health, Physical Education, Recreation, and Dance

1900 Association Drive, Reston, VA 20191, naspe@aahperd.org, 703-476-3410